GUIDELINES FOR
RAPID PARTICIPATORY APPRAISALS TO
ASSESS COMMUNITY HEALTH NEEDS

A Focus on Health Improvements for Low-Income
Urban and Rural Areas

by

Hugh Annett and Susan B. Rifkin

CONTENTS

Page

PREFACE

Despite continued national and international recognition of the plight of populations in underserved communities, especially in developing countries, inequity in health status not only continues to exist, but is increasing in most areas. Studies of health planning and decision-making show that health science and technology have not been widely applied to the advantage of low-income and poor populations in rural or urban areas.

To promote equity in health status and improve equitable access to health care, there is an urgent need to strengthen health planning for disadvantaged areas. This requires an assessment of the health status of deprived populations and their health problems, in order to determine priorities in health development and health services. These guidelines offer health managers a means of assessment, that is both rapid and involves the beneficiaries in the process of defining and addressing their own health needs, based on the principles of equity, participation and multisectoral cooperation.

The guidelines draw on the experiences of an urban primary health care project initiated, with assistance from the World Health Organization (WHO), in Tanga, United Republic of Tanzania by Dr H. Kasale, Medical Officer of Health, Tanga Municipal Authority. They were field-tested in Mbeya, United Republic of Tanzania, in collaboration with Mbeya Municipal Authority, and in Merseyside, England, where the South Sefton Health Authority used rapid appraisal to help restructure its work towards locality management.

The guidelines were first prepared in 1988 by Hugh Annett and Susan Rifkin, both at that time of the Department of International Community Health, Liverpool School of Tropical Medicine, Liverpool, England. Suggestions and comments made by various programmes in WHO headquarters, for which we were very grateful, were incorporated.

The original version of these guidelines was the outcome of support provided by the Swedish International Development Authority (SIDA), the Swedish Agency for Research Cooperation with Developing Countries (SAREC), and WHO collaboration with countries within the Organization's Programme for improving urban health.

The guidelines, which have been modified as a result of the field-testing, have a limited and specific application, as indicated in the text. Rapid appraisal is only one step in the planning process, and is confined to a participatory assessment of health needs, as perceived and defined by the community. However, health professionals have often commented on how this methodology has enabled them to discover "new" aspects of community life. In Mbeya, participants based in hospitals or training institutes gained significant insights into the problems of poor communities, while those working in the community discovered organizations and activities of which they had previously been unaware, so spreading knowledge and awareness across different levels. In Merseyside, rapid appraisal was used as a means of involving local people in planning and monitoring health interventions, as well as of developing and maintaining intersectoral multidisciplinary planning. The guidelines were also used at the training workshop on health systems reorientation in urban areas to reach the underserved, held in Lusaka, Zambia, in April 1989. Participants considered the guidelines to be an extremely important tool in helping the community to define its health needs and so contribute to its own health development. Health professionals, including planners, found rapid participatory appraisal a useful way of analysing current health activities, as well as a means of assessing health problems and their causes, leading to prioritization of health needs.

Since 1988, the guidelines have been used in a variety of urban and rural situations, both for training and for needs assessment, in developed and developing countries. Although reprinted, they are now again out of print. It has, therefore, been decided to amend and update them on the basis of experience gained in application, and to issue them once again, for wider use. It is hoped that they will assist health planners and decision-makers in formulating their health development programmes, and in allocating the required resources to the advantage of those who need, and should have equitable access to health care.

For their help in preparing the revision, acknowledgements are due to: Dr Scott Murray of the Department of General Practice, University of Edinburgh, Edinburgh, Scotland, Dr Corlien Varkevisser, Royal Tropical Institute, Amsterdam, Netherlands, Dr Wolfgang Bichmann, KfW, Frankfurt, Germany, and Korrie de Koning, Liverpool School of Tropical Medicine, Liverpool, England, all of whom have used and commented on the guidelines. We would also like to thank others, both students and practitioners, who have found the guidelines useful and, in some cases, even inspirational, and have given comments to help improve this revision. Sally Annett provided valuable assistance by reviewing the manuscript and making editorial corrections.

Dr I. Tabibzadeh
Chief, District Health Systems
Division of Strengthening of Health Services
World Health Organization
Geneva

CHAPTER 1. DEFINING RAPID PARTICIPATORY APPRAISAL

1.1 Introduction

How can health improvements be measured? In the past, because the improvements were presumed to be mainly a result of progress in biomedical technology and in service delivery, health status was seen as a sufficient measure. However, with the adoption of primary health care (PHC) by Member States of the World Health Organization (WHO) at Alma-Ata in 1978(*1*), it was recognized that good health is also influenced by socioeconomic conditions, and individual and community choices.

In order to understand what influences good health and how these influences work, WHO began to carry out country reviews of PHC. These reviews, undertaken by teams of nationals, WHO staff members and other agencies, have analysed changes in national health systems by examining national policies and programme developments, resources, health service coverage, and impact of health services, as well as processes of community involvement and of the search for equity. Lessons learned from these experiences are now being integrated into the development of district health programmes.

This document addresses two major concerns of WHO: determining the needs of the most vulnerable groups; and involving these groups in choices about their own health improvements. In this context, the challenge to health planners and managers is to work with these vulnerable communities to be able to describe the major threats to health, to set priorities for interventions to reduce these threats and to develop a plan of action based on these priorities. As there is little time and money available for the collection of the basic information needed to develop these plans, a method that provides comparatively rapid results, assessing both qualitative and quantitative aspects of health problems with minimum cost, is valuable.

One way of obtaining this information is to conduct a rapid appraisal in which health planners and managers review existing records, interview key informants and make observations, then together as a team, and with community participation, try to work out community priorities for action.

As explained later in section 1.2, rapid appraisal methodology is not new, nor is it the only methodology available for obtaining the information needed for planning. As a method for improving health, however, it not only benefits from a fairly quick and cost-effective approach, but it also strengthens the PHC principles of equity, participation, and multisectoral cooperation. In terms of equity, it focuses on members of society who are still denied the benefits to which they are legally entitled and which are received by more affluent members of society. As regards participation, it uses key informants (members of the community who, because of their official or unofficial leadership positions, represent a wide range of community views) both to identify community problems and to contribute to solutions. In terms of a multisectoral approach, it uses those responsible for the allocation of resources, such as health staff, sanitary and water engineers, social workers and financial planners, to do the investigations and to draw up a plan of action to address priority problems.

The methodology presented here, entitled rapid participatory appraisal (RPA), is only the first step in the process of formulating a plan of action. Further steps are briefly discussed and reference is made to documents where details may be found. This step, however, is perhaps the most crucial, since it involves gathering information and developing mechanisms to obtain and act upon this information. By taking professionals with a range of expertise to address health problems, by involving community members in defining and suggesting solutions to these problems, and by using the method as the means to develop, not merely the end of, an action programme for health improvements, RPA provides the opportunity to lay a strong foundation for the PHC approach to improving health in low-income areas.

1.2   Background

Rapid appraisal, as its name implies, is a method to enable planners to obtain information quickly and, in terms of time and monetary expenditure, relatively cheaply. It was first promoted as a planning method in the late 1970s. It began in the field of rural development, focusing on farming systems research, but expanded rapidly to other areas, including health and nutrition. The evolution of rapid appraisal is reflected in the variety of names given to various adaptations. The approach developed here is known as **rapid participatory appraisal** and is defined in section 1.4. The name is not chosen to confuse people further about the method, but rather to distinguish it from the other approaches described below and summarized in the box on page 14.

Rapid appraisal, as a planning concept was developed by Chambers and a group of colleagues at the Institute of Development Studies in Sussex, England, with a view to improving planning in the field of agriculture and rural development in developing countries(2). Named *rapid rural appraisal*, it sought to overcome the barriers of:
(1) undertaking long surveys, the result of which came too late for use in planning; and
(2) the biases of planning experts who travelled paved roads in the dry season, talked to elite groups, and designed programmes after only limited access to the majority of proposed beneficiaries. Because planners spent time with some of the poorest rural people, involved them in the data collection process and discussed problems mutually identified by planners and local people, rapid rural appraisal was seen as a means of addressing the problems of the poor by obtaining quick and accurate information to identify these problems and taking relatively immediate action to solve them.

Rapid rural appraisal quickly went beyond the mere interaction of planners with local people, to active participation of communities. This expansion into *participatory rural appraisal* has focused on the development of techniques involving the community as partners in information collection and analysis and the decision-making process(4,5).

2

These two approaches rest on two principles(6):

(1)   optimal ignorance, which demands that information that is not relevant to the objectives of the collection exercise must be ignored;

(2)   proportionate accuracy, which demands that the accuracy of information should be kept in proportion to its use, and that time should not be "wasted" in validating information that serves no applicable purpose.

The characteristics of rapid rural appraisal and participatory rural appraisal are:

-       collection of action-oriented information to be used by planners and managers for problem-solving;

-       community involvement in information collection and analysis;

-       emphasis on communication and listening skills;

-       reinterpretation of hypothesis as more information becomes available (iterative approach);

-       holistic approach to data interpretation;

-       use of mulitidisciplinary teams of professionals.

In the field of health and nutrition, rapid appraisals were first used in the 1980s. An early approach was *rapid epidemiological assessment*, which is rooted in the disciplines of epidemiology and statistics, and which consists of rapid data collection through small area survey and sampling, surveillance methods, screening and individual risk assessment, and community indicators of risk or health status(7). It has mainly been used to evaluate health service functioning where constraints on staff time are critical.

Rapid assessment procedures, also a product of the 1980s, are grounded in the discipline of medical anthropology. They have been used to gain community and target group views about the causes of and cures for poor health, and reactions to specific health interventions. The approach emphasizes the use of anthropological techniques for information collection on community health and nutrition situations. The techniques are specifically aimed at gaining information about views and beliefs about health, the treatment and prevention of disease, and the use of both traditional and modern health care. A training manual based on the use of these methods in 16 countries has been produced(8).

Closely related to this approach in its use of anthropological techniques is *rapid ethnographic assessment(9)*. Emerging from experience with rapid assessment procedures, it uses the same techniques but focuses on the collection of data concerning beliefs and practices in relation to specific diseases. Under the auspices of WHO, this approach has been used, for example, to improve management of acute respiratory infections(*10*).

Rapid assessment procedures and rapid ethnographic assessment both rely on traditional anthropological techniques, including individual and group interviews, observations and use of existing documents. These qualitative techniques are also used by practitioners of rapid rural appraisal/participatory rural appraisal.

Types of rapid appraisals

Rapid rural appraisal

Multidisciplinary teams collect data from people in the community. Orginally used in the areas of agriculture and rural development

Participatory rural appraisal

An extension of rapid rural appraisal in which planners and the community are partners in information collection and analysis and proposed actions

Rapid epidemiological assessment

Surveys, sampling and risk assessments are undertaken to evaluate health service functions

Rapid assessment procedures

Anthropological methods are used to assess community views of health and diseases and health interventions

Rapid ethnographic assessment

Anthropological methods are used to assess community beliefs and practices in relation to specific disease interventions

---

Rapid appraisals share a number of characteristics. They:

- are relatively quick and cheap carry out;
- address the problems of communities rather than individuals, usually poor communities;
- provide information for action rather than research;
- recognize that the approach is not static, but is changing and evolving new techniques.

However, the rapid appraisals developed in the areas of agricultural and rural development areas differ in two significant ways from those which responded mainly to health and nutrition problems. They:

-   seek to involve local people in the appraisal process not only to extract information from them;

-   rely on multidisciplinary teams and approaches for information collection and analysis, rather than teams from just one discipline, e.g., epidemiology or anthropology.

In the period since these rapid appraisals were first formulated, their application has quickly expanded. Already in the 1980s, groups were combining the health and nutrition approaches with those from rural development to ensure a wider understanding and a more solid base for programme planning. The three boxes below illustrate some published examples of these combined appraisals.

**Rapid assessment of community nutrition problems
in Parbhani, India**

Undertaken with the support of the International Development Research Centre of Canada, the objective of this assessment was to investigate the cause of malnutrition in the western dry land region of India(11). Combining qualitative methods to involve community people in the appraisal and quantitative methods to address the magnitude of the problem, information was gathered through open-ended surveys, in-depth interviews and discussions with local people to discover food habits and beliefs. This was supplemented with secondary information on health facilities, food distribution systems and nutrient supplementation programmes. On the basis of the information collected, recommendations were formulated concerning further research, policy changes, market strategies and wider participation of local groups in the programme.

**Rapid appraisal of health and nutrition in
a PHC project in Pahou, Benin**

Jointly implemented by the Centre Régional pour le Développement de la Santé (PDS), Benin and the Royal Tropical Institute, Amsterdam, Netherlands, the aim of this project was to propose health and nutrition interventions that could be undertaken to improve the health and nutrition of mothers and children in three zones in South Benin(12). Combining quantitative survey techniques for sampling and for describing the magnitude of the problem of malnutrition and qualitative methods for interviewing mothers on possible causes, multidisciplinary teams developed the analytical framework and undertook data collection techniques, and did the data collection and analysis together. Their reports were fed back to those in the village that participated in the study. The amount of information gathered allowed programme proposals to be formulated and adopted. The validity of the information was confirmed by an extensive epidemiological socioeconomic and nutritional survey undertaken shortly afterwards.

**Rapid appraisal to assess urban community
health needs in Mbeya, United Republic of Tanzania and in the United Kingdom**

The appraisal in Mbeya was supported by WHO(13). A team composed of officials from a variety of divisions within the municipal authority's office undertook the appraisal in the context of a 10-day workshop facilitated by the authors of this document. The exercise became the basis for the original edition of these guidelines(14). The participants in the workshop began by determining what information was needed, the people who might best give information, and the types of observations and secondary data necessary to cross-check information from interviews. Field work was undertaken to collect the data, which were then analysed by the team, who returned subsequently to the interviewees to confirm information and to prioritize the problems identified. The result was a draft plan of action to improve health conditions in three lower-income wards in the town.

One other outcome of this appraisal was that the guidelines stimulated individuals and health authorities in the United Kingdom to use this approach to assess health needs in their locality(15). More recently, it has become even more popular as general practitioners in the United Kingdom have become fund holders for the services they provide and, therefore, must have some basis for deciding how to allocate money. It appeals to those practitioners in low-income areas who are committed to providing the best service for the most number of people(16).

1.3   Purpose of the document

The purpose of this document is to provide health planners and managers with guidelines for undertaking a needs assessment in poor communities with the involvement of the people in those communities. The guidelines describe in detail the steps necessary to make the assessment and highlight the basic skills needed and methods used. In addition, examples of this type of assessment are presented.

To supplement the text, annexes provide outlines for workshops to implement the assessment and detailed suggestions about appropriate questions. In addition, an annotated bibliography lists easily obtainable publications that provide more detailed information concerning skills, methods and experiences related to this type of appraisal.

It is hoped that this revised version responds both to new developments in the field and to comments from those have used the original guidelines.

1.4   What is rapid participatory appraisal?

Rapid participatory appraisal (RPA) is a method for obtaining information about a set of problems in a short period, without a large expenditure of professional time and finances, and with involvement of community members. It is employed as a way of assessing needs prior to the preparation of plans for future action, and is thus the first step in the planning process.

As described in these guidelines, RPA can be used to assess community health needs as a first step in planning health interventions for specific communities. The aim is to involve those who are the less advantaged in determining their own health needs and, together with the health managers who have resources to meet those needs (government authorities and nongovernmental organizations), in taking action to solve the problems identified.

> Rapid participatory appraisal is a way of collecting the information needed for formulating a plan of action. It is not a method for collecting extensive data on one geographical area or one particular health problem.

The term "rapid" refers both to the time spent in the field collecting the data and the time spent analysing the data. This should be the minimum acceptable time needed to gather the information required for developing a plan of action. Rapid appraisals have been seen by many to be similar to an exercise to produce a simple map of a particular geographical area. They help to describe the main features, such as the hills, rivers and valleys, but they do not provide details, such as how high the hills are, or how deep the rivers and valleys.

> Rapid participatory appraisal indicates what the problems are not how many people are affected by them.

> Rapid participatory appraisal is:
>
> - a means of obtaining information in a short period of time without a large expenditure of money and professional time
> - a step in the planning process
> - a method of rapid analysis
> - a methodology for participation

RPA rests on three principles(3).

1. **Collect only relevant and necessary data** because this is the only way in which a rapid assessment can be made. Data should not be collected because they are easily available, or because they might eventually be used. It is self-defeating if data are collected quickly but are so extensive that they take a long time to analyse.

2.   **Decide what information is needed and find acceptable ways of obtaining it.**
While information may be directly abstracted from written documents, other ways
must be found to gain information from people. When it is not possible to obtain
information by asking a direct question, it may be necessary to ask a substitute
question or make an observation as a "proxy" for a direct question. The most
striking example of this use of proxy information is in assessing family income,
particularly in low-income areas where there is high unemployment and wages are
non-existent. A proxy question such as, "What is the household expenditure?" or,
"What type of material is used to build the accommodation?" or, "What kinds and
numbers of meals do family members have?", might have to be used as an
indicator of family income.

Involve the community in the rapid appraisal exercise. Experience in low-
income areas has indicated the need to extend this principle. The community must
be involved in defining its own problems and seeking relevant solutions, not merely
in providing information for planners to use in gaining acceptance of a predeter-
mined health intervention. Where programmes - mostly on a small scale - have
been successful, it has been where the people and decision-makers together
planned steps for community health improvements. Banerji(17) discusses in detail
how this approach allowed Indian planners to gain acceptance of their programmes
for tuberculosis. Others have described how needs-based planning has led to
relatively cost-effective, self-sustaining programmes(18). Among poverty stricken
people, where resources are scarce and land security and income are tenuous,
interventions that do not gain the support of those who can benefit are likely to be
at best misused, at worst ignored.

Principles of RPA

1.   Do not collect too much or irrelevant data.
2.   Adjust investigations to reflect local conditions and specific situations.
3.   Involve community people in both defining community needs and seeking possible solutions.

To achieve the objectives of RPA, investigators must have the necessary attitudes
and skills: the determination to find and follow, and then examine critically the existing
written record; the willingness to learn from local people and use indigenous resources;
the ability to listen carefully during interviews and informal conversations; the capacity to
keep a sharp eye open and to observe the surroundings for clues about problems and
potential solutions. To these four can be added a fifth: the ability to use common sense
in analysing the information. If the conclusions do not reflect their professional knowledge
and experience, the investigators should probably review their interpretation of the data.

1.5 Using pictures to present information - the information pyramid

An important aspect of rapid appraisals, particularly in the rural development sector, has been the introduction of pictures (frequently in the form of diagrams) when collecting and interpreting information. A visual presentation helps the members of a team to understand each other when they have different professional backgrounds, and to understand community contributors. Some of the more innovative pictures and their contribution to the appraisal process will be introduced in Chapter 3.

One type of picture, which has proved particularly useful for RPAs to assess community health needs is the information pyramid. It provides a checklist for asking questions and a framework for analysis, and so forms **the basis of an approach for obtaining and analysing data that will enable planners to have useful, although not exhaustive, information with which to identify the health problems of people living in a defined geographical area and seek solutions.**

Information pyramids have three characteristics:

- they are based on needs identified by the community;

- they are built on information gathered from documents, from a dialogue between planners and community members, and from the observations of planners in the community;

- they are constructed in the recognition that communities often experience comparatively rapid change and, therefore, that the pyramids reflect the situation only at a given point in time - the information in a pyramid changes as information is gathered at various points in time.

An example of an information pyramid for assessing community needs with a view to planning interventions for health improvements is shown in Figure I and described below.

Figure I   **Blocks for an information pyramid for use in assesssing community health needs**

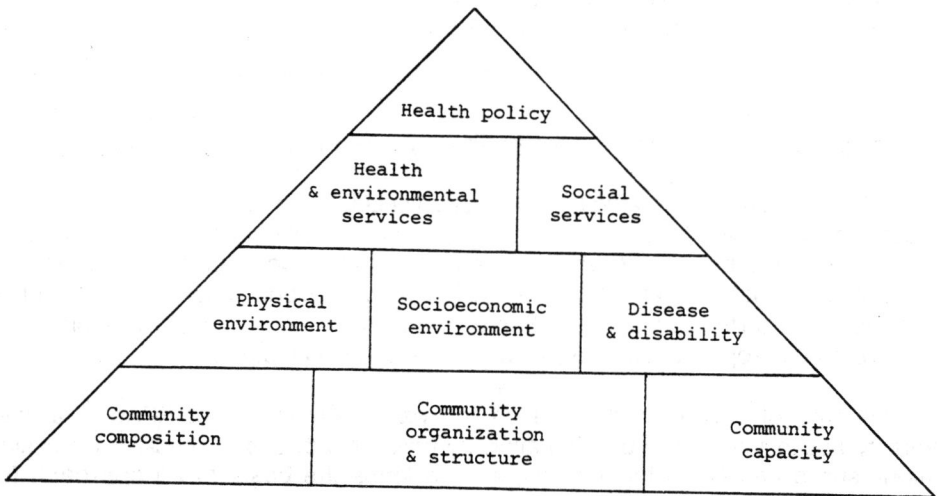

```
                            Health policy

                     Health
                 & environmental      Social
                    services         services

          Physical        Socioeconomic      Disease
         environment       environment     & disability

    Community           Community              Community
    composition         organization           capacity
                        & structure
```

The pyramid is built on a foundation of information about community composition, organization and capacities to act. Health planners and managers need to know about the community with which they are working and to discover the strengths and weaknesses of the community leadership, organizations and structures.

The next level of the pyramid describes the socioecological factors that influence health, including the physical environment, socioeconomic conditions and disease and disability. This information is needed to investigate the potentials for and barriers to community improvements. Data on the physical environment are used to determine the environmental causes of disease and disability. Data on social aspects focus on traditional beliefs and values that facilitate or impede behavioural changes. An analysis of economic aspects highlights income sources, earning potential and the economic opportunities of various community groups.

The third level concerns data on the existence, coverage, accessibility and acceptability of services including health services, environmental services such as water and waste disposal, and social services such as education and assistance for the disabled.

At the top of the pyramid, the final level, for which some general knowledge is required, concerns national, regional and local policies about health improvements for low-income areas. Information on these policies, particularly health policies, will indicate whether the political leadership is committed to primary health care. With strong government support at both the top and local levels, health improvements for the urban and rural poor will have the potential to proceed more rapidly, and without major political barriers.

When planners undertake RAPs to plan for health improvements, they collect blocks of information relating to these four general levels and so build up the pyramid. Its shape reminds them that success depends on building a planning process that rests on a strong community information base, and that the amount of information needed about each area is relative to its position on the pyramid. It is the quality of the information not the quantity that is most crucial.

Using the information pyramid

An information pyramid provides the framework, in picture form, for the collection and analysis of data. To reinforce this visual method of presenting data, RPA teams use paper of three different colours (in constructing the pyramid), for example, blue paper for information from interviews, green paper for information from observations, and yellow paper for information from documents. Scrap paper can be used (A4 size cut into three or four equal parts). In deciding what information is to be collected, team members use felt pens to write down key words on the blank paper (e.g. "water sources", "main income", "main diseases"), the colour of which indicates where such information can be obtained. For this example, "water sources" is written on a green paper; "income sources" is written on blue paper; "major diseases" is written on yellow paper. These papers are then placed in the block of the pyramid that defines the category to which each idea belongs. When this exercise is complete, a checklist of information is created.

When analysing the information obtained from the field work, the same process is used. Key words are written upon paper, the colour of which corresponds to the source of the information, then placed in the block on the pyramid corresponding to the general category to which the information belongs.

Used in this fashion, the pyramid:

- allows teams to see, in picture form, whether there is any imbalance in the information that is due to be or has been collected;
- provides categories both for collection and for analysis of information;
- enables teams to see whether information has come from more than one source (triangulation) and has thus been cross-checked.

CHAPTER 2. CONDUCTING RAPID PARTICIPATORY APPRAISALS

2.1   Preparation

Rapid appraisal is a team exercise and one that is carried out in the field. The team should consist of people who are responsible for resources to support interventions and who have a wide range of professional skills and expertise. These people will be representing their professions, as well as the municipal authorities. In the urban setting, for example, the health problems of low-income groups need to be solved by health staff, sanitary engineers, architects, social workers and municipal financial officers, among others. In a rural setting, team members might include the provincial/district medical officer, the water engineer, the education officer, community development staff, agricultural officers and members of nongovernmental organizations working in the area of social development.

For identifying health problems in low-income areas, RPA is best undertaken by a multisectoral team comprising those who are responsible for the resources necessary to help solve the problems found.

An RPA can be carried out by bringing the team together for a 10-day workshop. The workshop should be facilitated by at least one person who has had experience in rapid appraisal, whose role is to serve as a focal point for decisions and facilitate the discussions. The steps followed are presented in section 2.2.

The collection and analysis of the required data occupy the workshop participants for five or six days. The concluding sessions of the workshop should focus on using the results of the RPA to draw up and implement a plan of action. A suitable timetable for such a workshop is given in Annex 1.

In some situations, however, it may be impractical to set aside a 10-day period for the conduct of the RPA. An alternative is to hold an introductory three-day workshop, and to fit the data collection into the normal working schedule of the investigators over the following two to three weeks, or over the following few months. Once data collection is complete, a concluding workshop of two days will be necessary to complete data analysis and prepare a plan of action. This approach is more difficult to manage than an intensive 10-day workshop but it can still be a very useful exercise. A possible timetable for this second option is given in Appendix 2.

2.2 Steps for a rapid participatory appraisal

RPAs are conducting following a series of steps, which are listed in the box and described in detail below. It is important to remember that the appraisal is the first step in the planning process, and that data collection is not an end in itself.

Summary of steps for a rapid participatory appraisal

1. Define rapid participatory appraisal.

2. Decide what information is needed.

3. Decide how to obtain information

   - key informant interviews;
   - observations;
   - documents.

4. Collect information.

5. Analyse information
   - data and professional "common sense".

6. Review findings with key informants.

7. Define priorities.

8. Prepare the final report.

2.2.1 Step one. Define rapid participatory appraisal

Before the team begins the RPA all the members should understand and share its objectives. One contribution to this process is defining the terms; Chapter 1 is designed as the basis for this introduction. Another contribution is for the team members to share their expectations of the exercise. The facilitator might ask each team member to write down expectations and present them to the group. A third, and the most critical contribution is learning communication and listening skills. These skills are discussed in more detail in Chapter 3.

2.2.2 Step two. Decide what information is needed

The decisions about what information is to be obtained, how it is to be collected, and the exact questions to be asked must be made locally by each team, depending on the amount of information already available and on the local conditions. It is not possible to develop a universal checklist. As already stressed, RPA is part of the planning process, and thus is reflective of the process in a specific situation.

The information pyramid described in section 1.3 provides a framework for deciding what information is needed. General guidance on possible areas for information collection, in particular in relation to problems in poor communities, and their importance is given in Annex 3. While it may not be possible to collect information about each of these areas, the list provided may prove useful in:

- serving as a basis for the development of an interview protocol, and for determining which data can be extracted from written records;

- reminding the team about areas on which information might be usefully recorded as observations;

- aiding the interpretation of the information collected.

2.2.3 Step three. Decide how to obtain the information

Rapid appraisals depend on triangulation (cross-checking) of data to ensure scientific rigour. In other words, information must be confirmed either by asking several people from different backgrounds the same question, or by obtaining information from more than one source. The major sources of information are interviews with key informants by team members, and reports and other documents.

Key informants. Key informants are people in the community who, because of their official position or informal leadership, have access to information about community, rather than individual, views about community problems. For this reason, they can be seen as representatives of a range of opinions held by the community. The people selected will vary, according to the specific situation and the purpose of the RPA. A suggested list is summarized in the box and described briefly below.

Information can be obtained from key informants in a number of ways. Skills and methods for interviewing are described in Chapter 3.

```
┌─────────────────────────────────────────────────────────────────────┐
│                          Key informants                              │
│                                                                       │
│   Government officials                                                │
│   Social and health service personnel                                │
│   Traditional healers                                                 │
│   Teachers                                                            │
│   Community leaders:    - elected officials                           │
│                         - heads of community organizations            │
│                         - religious leaders                           │
│                         - women's group leaders                       │
│                         - informal leaders.                           │
│   Owners of local shops and entertainment establishments             │
│   Members of nongovernmental organizations working in the area        │
│                                                                       │
│   Remember! This list may be modified depending on each specific situation │
└─────────────────────────────────────────────────────────────────────┘
```

Government officials. Government authorities are important sources of information on major health issues, and on policy options that deal with these issues. They also have information on communities marked for special attention. While some officers may be members of the investigation team, those whose departments are not represented can be interviewed. The information and experience provided by government officials in the planning stages is crucial, because these people will be involved in subsequent programme development.

Social and health service personnel. The staff in charge of governmental and nongovernmental organization facilities and community projects are sources of data not only on their own services, but also on the activities of other service providers, traditional and private, in the vicinity. Staff actually working in and with the community are the prime source of data. Supervisory or managerial staff removed from the field can provide data on community-wide problems, and on inter-community comparisons. Those involved in enforcing legislation, social workers and health inspectors, can provide data on the benefits or lack of benefits under the law, as well as information about the inadequacies of legislation. Others who can provide information include private medical practitioners. A sympathetic private practitioner will be a good source of data on the services provided, clients served, standards maintained and fees charged in private health care facilities.

Traditional healers. A knowledgeable traditional practitioner is an invaluable source of data on the numbers of traditional practitioners in a community, level of community use and the rates of remuneration.

Teachers. As a particular category of social sector personnel, teachers are important informants because of their intimate contact with both children and parents in the community. If children travel outside the community to schools, then the teachers responsible for these children should also be interviewed. In poor areas, official educational facilities may not be available. In these situations, volunteers who run informal schooling or crèches can often be useful sources of information.

Community leaders. Community leaders and representatives can be sources of data on a wide range of subjects. Those in official positions can provide an overall view about the community and its problems. They can also help to identify others who can provide more specific information. However, formal leaders, usually men, often present views that do not necessarily represent all their constituents. Politically, they may tend to favour those to whom they owe their position, often the economically advantaged members of the community and it could be misleading to rely solely on what they say about vulnerable groups, including women and the poorest of the poor. It is therefore important to interview representatives of vulnerable sections of the community, in order to learn directly about their concerns and needs. Other informants include the officials of organizations that operate in the community, leaders of religious groups and the heads of women's organizations. These leaders provide insights into the specific groups they represent, as well as the problems of these groups within the community as a whole. Also, informal leaders who have been identified during the interviews of influential people are often very good sources of information.

Owners of local shops and entertainment establishments. These informants are important because they are in contact with a broad range of inhabitants in the area. They hear of and see problems which may not, for various reasons, come to the ears of the formal leadership, also escaping recognition by those in more specialized services. Although the information these people provide might be more difficult to analyse, it might also be very valuable as a means of identifying problems overlooked by other groups.

Members of nongovernmental organizations working in the area. Although people attached to these organizations are usually not community residents, their work in the community gives them a knowledge and concern that is very valuable for assessing community problems and needs. Those in organizations with a narrow focus, such as tuberculosis control, may have only a limited vision. Others, particularly those concerned with community development, can provide an overview of the community rarely found in other key informants. They may also prove willing allies in the planning process, providing human and material resources to undertake community improvement programmes.

Observations. Observations on the environment in which the RPA is being conducted are an important aspect of data collection. They may cover problems not specifically discussed with or overlooked by key informants, and may confirm or contradict the information provided by them. The ways in which observations can be made are discussed in section 3.3.

Observations should be recorded by team members and compared with those of other team members during data analysis. The team can use its professional experience to evaluate these observations and determine how they might be included in the final report. Important observations should be discussed with key informants during the second round of interviews.

Reports and other documents. Although written records do have limitations, they are still an important source of information. They also provide a start for building an information pyramid. Records that might prove useful are listed in the box. However, it is quite likely that others are available and known to the planning team. The team must continually remember that the purpose of RPA is to get relevant information quickly. Substantial documents may contain only a limited amount of relevant information; they should be purposefully scanned for that information rather than read in detail.

Sources of written information

Census statistics.
Planning records.
Accounts showing budgetary expenditures.
Reports of surveys that have already been undertaken.
Reports of studies undertaken at local universities.
Historical records.
Hospital and clinic records.
Reports of studies undertaken by international agencies.
Reports of surveys undertaken by nongovernmental organizations.
Ministry records, i.e. relating to health, housing, environmental
  sanitation, water, social services, and city plans.

2.2.4 Step four. Collect the information

Once the team has decided how to collect the information, and detailed by name the key informants to be interviewed, preparations for the field work can be begin. Before actual field work gets under way, it is important to pilot test the questions; a half-day pilot study among groups of people similar to those who will be interviewed is useful. Pilot testing indicates questions that are unclear, that get a response different to that anticipated, or that are difficult for respondents to answer. In addition, it allows the team to estimate how long it will take each key informant to answer the questions, and to see how the work might be divided, and which team member might be responsible for what task. Team members will also have an opportunity to test their skills in conducting semi-structured interviews. They can help each other to become aware of willingness to learn from local people, to listen to formal answers and informal conversations, and to observe their surroundings.

Pilot testing: An example

The members of a planning team in a municipality developed a list of questions, then field tested them in three different low-income urban settlements. One question attempted to assess income in order to identify poorer members of the community. When key informants were asked how many people were very poor, they always gave one or more names of "poor" individuals but they were unable to conceptually find a criterion for identifying the poorest. As a result, the attempt had to be abandoned and the team had to rely on reports and on observations to assess poverty levels.

Once pilot testing has been completed, the team is ready to undertake the field study. It is useful to split the team into smaller groups in order to cover a larger area and more people. Experience suggests that groups of three people are suitable. While one person is pursuing a line of enquiry, another can be taking notes and a third preparing the next set of questions. Team members should change roles during the interview to allow each to ask questions in the area of his or her professional expertise.

2.2.5 Step five. Analyse the information

Most of the data collected in the interviews, by observation and from documents is in the form of statements, opinions, descriptions - none of which are readily quantified. It is more difficult to process such qualitative data and it is, therefore, all the more important to approach it in a systematic fashion. The procedure can be divided into three phases:

- identifying categories;
- sorting answers;
- interpreting findings.

As indicated in section 1.5, the information pyramid can be used as an aid in this process.

First, information from key informant interviews should be compared with information obtained from the review of secondary documents, and from observations. If there are large discrepancies in the sets of data, the areas of difference should be noted and a decision taken about how to validate the findings. At this point, the team might decide to undertake a more intensive survey to confirm one set of findings (see section 2.2.8).

Next, the data in each category should be summarized to produce a concise statement of the main findings for each question. These summaries should be reviewed and discussed by the whole team. Once confirmed in this way, they can be grouped into the blocks of the information pyramid. The information pyramid then forms the basis for the team's final report.

Finally, the team uses the findings, the observations and the professional knowledge of its members to make a list of the major problems in the community surveyed. This list may well include problems that the professionals identified, but community members did not. Whether these problems are important to people in the community is validated in the next step.

2.2.6 Step 6. Review information with key informants

Team members next return to the key informants to ask their opinion about the priority they place upon the different problems defined during data analysis. This approach is based on a modified Delphi method[1]. One way in which this can be done is to write each problem on a separate sheet of paper, and ask key informants to arrange the papers in order of priority. This was the method adopted in the example shown in the box. If a problem has been identified by the team which is not seen as a problem by community leaders, it will be given low priority in this priority-setting exercise.

Reviewing information

The members of an appraisal team analysed the data they had collected, and identified problems for the squatter areas where they were conducting their investigation. They then arranged to return to the field to review the findings with key informants. Each of the eight problems was written down on a separate card. Key informants were given the eight cards and asked to arrange them in order of priority. These rankings were scored, giving a score of eight to the problem given the top priority, a score of seven to the problem in second place and so on. Taking the scores from all the key informants, an average score for each problem was calculated, to give an overall list of priorities.

2.2.7 Step seven. Define priorities

The team is now ready to seek solutions to the problems identified taking into account the priorities indicated by key informants. During interviews, key informants will no doubt have expressed some ideas about how to tackle the problems. In addition, team members will also have ideas related to the resources available through their own departments. Team members must now decide which interventions they are prepared to undertake.

---

[1]   The term derives from the oracle who lived in Delphi, in ancient Greece, forecasting the future.

Practitioners of rapid appraisal in the rural sector have suggested that this step can be accomplished by developing a feasibility matrix(19). In the context of health improvements, each intervention can be examined for the following characteristics:

- health benefit (what is the overall health impact?);

- community capacity for self-help (how committed is the community to solving the problems and what can it contribute to their solution?);

- sustainability (can the intervention be maintained and at what cost?);

- equity (which income groups are likely to benefit most?);

- cost (what are the initial capital and staff costs?);

- time for benefit (how long will it be before changes are noticeable?).

The table below shows the feasibility matrix prepared for priority-setting during the RPA conducted in Mbeya, United Republic of Tanzania, mentioned in Chapter 1. Analysis of the data collected revealed a number of problems for which interventions were suggested. Each intervention was assessed in terms of the criteria listed above and the results were entered in the matrix. It was recommended that highest priority should be given to undertaking the intervention with the highest feasibility score.

Recommendation/ Innovation	Health benefit	Capacity for self-help/ participation	Sustain-ability	Equity	Cost	Time for benefit	Feasibility score	Priority
1. Every house to have a latrine built by the family	+ + +	+ +	+ + +	+ + +	+	+	13	(2)
2. Provision of roads	+ + +	+ + +	+	+ +	+	+	11	(3)
3. Construct refuse bays and institute garbage collection	+ + +	+ + +	+ +	+ + +	+	+ + +	15	(1)

Each intervention is scored by giving "+" for low, "+ +" for medium and "+ + +" for high value. The one with the highest total score (feasibility score) is given the highest priority.

2.2.8 Step eight. Prepare the final report

Information needs to be shared both with those who participated in the appraisal and with a wider community of interested people. This can be done by writing and presenting a final report of the RPA, which should consist of:

-   an introduction and overview of the community/area under study;

-   a review of major problems in the community/area;

-   the findings of the RPA based on key informant interviews, observations and the documents review;

-   recommendations.

A short summary of the findings and an outline of the implications of these findings for future action should make up the main body of the document. These are based on the information pyramid constructed during data analysis, and on the feasibility matrix for priority-setting. The details of the interviews and the final summaries can be provided as annexes.

The report should be made available to all those who participated in the interviews. If funds are not sufficient to send each informant a copy of the report, a one-page summary can be sent, together with details of where a full report can be seen.

Credibility and cooperation for the future programme depends on feedback. Provide all key informants with a report of the RPA or at least an executive summary.

2.3   Using the results

The report of the RPA becomes the basis for the next phase in the planning process. This phase begins by calling together members of the RPA team and a small number of key informants to review the findings of the report, and suggest future actions.

2.3.1 Preparing a plan of action and setting specific objectives

There are several methods available for preparing a plan of action. While it is not possible to review alternatives here, the purpose of the entire exercise is the use of a PHC approach to improve the health of poor urban and rural communities, and the RPA technique in which key informants identify problems is the method used to make the community needs assessment; participatory planning approaches involving both resource holders and the people in the community are therefore again recommended. An example of the type of methodology, has been published by Deutsche Gesellschaft für Technische Zuammenarbeit [German Technical Development Agency](20). Involvement of the community in planning will promote a sense of ownership of the future programme, encouraging compliance with suggested actions and contributions towards costs.

At the end of this step, the team should set specific objectives, setting a schedule for meeting objectives and designating a responsible person for each activity. A logical framework or matrix might be useful to assist the team in this endeavour.

One objective may well be to obtain more detailed information about a specific problem. This would probably require the collection of quantitative information, since at this stage of the planning process, it becomes necessary to know not merely what the problems are, but how big they are. In other words, it is now time to obtain a good approximation of how many people are affected by this problem, and what resources are available in local authorities, the community and nongovernmental organizations, for solving it.

A detailed survey is more useful at this point in the planning process, than as a preliminary step. It can be targeted on priority problems defined by the RPA, so that a more limited survey is required, which can be conducted more quickly and with less resources than would otherwise be the case. Furthermore, following its involvement in the RPA, the community will be more inclined to recognize the importance of information for planning, and be more prepared to give its support to the survey.

Such a survey can be included as an early activity in the development of a plan of action. This strategy will enable project funds to be allocated for the survey, which might otherwise not be feasible on financial grounds.

Planners can draw on a range of techniques for defining major health problems, including standard epidemiological sample surveys and case studies. For estimating childhood mortality, for example, a number of new methods are now available for use where vital registration and census data are inadequate(23). The annotated bibliography at the end of this document indicates sources to guide planners in this activity.

2.3.2 Monitoring and evaluation

Monitoring and evaluation are closely related, but distinct activities(24); they have different purposes, and usually involve different people:

- **Monitoring** is an internal project activity which enables managers to implement a project in an efficient manner. It involves review and surveillance of project implementation, to ensure that it is proceeding according to plan;

- **Evaluation** examines more fundamental questions concerning the continuing relevance of a project and the appropriateness of its objectives and strategies in the light of experience; evaluation usually involves individuals not directly concerned with project implementation.

Because the process of designing and implementing health development projects is complex, the results and impact of many of them have been disappointing. Monitoring and evaluation provide an opportunity for learning from and improving a project as it proceeds; they are essential components in the implementation of a project, and can be key factors in its success. Provision for monitoring and evaluation should therefore be included in the plan of action.

Monitoring and evaluation are learning processes for all those involved in a project and should therefore be as participatory as possible(25). Involving community representatives can lead to a better understanding of these processes, an awareness of the constraints, and continued participation and support for the project.

Monitoring and evaluation involve the use of indicators to measure, or "indicate" changes in a situation. The selection of useful indicators is not easy, and requires that the objectives of the plan of action, or project, are specific and stated with clarity. A plan of action need not prescribe indicators in detail, but should provide suggestions on key aspects to be monitored: the results of the RPA can be used to identify these. Indicators must also be kept to a minimum otherwise the collection and processing of the data, both qualitative and quantitative, required can consume an excessive amount of resources. The information generated by the RPA, and by the baseline survey if one is included in a plan of action, provides useful reference material for the subsequent monitoring and evaluation of a project.

CHAPTER 3. SKILLS AND METHODS FOR
DATA COLLECTION

3.1 Communication skills

As indicated in the previous chapter, key informant interviews are one of the three sources of information for RPAs. The success of interviewing depends on good communication. Two skills critical to achieving this goal are listening and facilitating dialogues; the first skill is the basis of the second.

Listening, in this case, means hearing what is being said, not what the interviewer wants to hear. This skill is not easy to acquire; experience is the best route to proficiency, although participation in exercises that reveal individual strengths and weaknesses is useful at the outset. RPA teams should therefore spend at least one day undertaking a series of exercises, which include role play and self-analysis, to become aware of their own listening abilities. A book by Johnston and Rifkin (see annotated bibliography, section 4) provides a number of examples of this type of exercise, as well as exercises for developing skills in facilitating discussions, in team work and in leadership, and could be used as a manual for team training for community interaction.

The members of the team must all act as facilitators, both in the information collection and in building consensus for action with community leaders. Facilitating skills can also be learned by raising awareness of personal weaknesses, and with practice, and it is well worth setting aside some time for this purpose. Careful listening is the basis, but skills must also be acquired to enable interviewers to ask clear questions, rephrase obscure ideas and summarize main discussion points. Team members must also be able to create an atmosphere of mutual exchange, rather than of domination by either the professionals or a strong and outspoken key informant.

> RPA team members must listen carefully and must not offer their own views. Any judgement will hinder the flow of information and bring bias to the findings.

Listening and facilitating dialogue are tools for building mutual respect between the team and key informants. The participatory dimension of an appraisal is based on this concept. In the past, professionals have often used their position and power to manipulate beneficiaries into accepting what the professionals have decided is best. It is particularly important for the team to be aware of the community's previous experiences and how these have shaped expectations. A conscious effort must be made to overcome this legacy, and to build relationships where both planners and people in the community recognize the important contribution each makes to solving mutually identified problems.

3.2. Conducting interviews

3.2.1 Semi-structured interviews

In order to get good information from key informants, the RPA team needs, in addition to communication skills, a systematic approach to the interview situation. In this section, ways in which this approach can be developed are suggested.

The basis of information collection from key informants, both as individuals and in groups, is the semi-structured interview, which is a guided discussion conducted in a manner that is sufficiently informal to encourage the informant to introduce subjects or aspects of subjects not anticipated by the interviewer. This type of interview is the most appropriate for RPA, as the topics on which data are being sought are complex, requiring qualitative rather than quantitative answers.

Good practices will ensure that semi-structured interviews are productive. The most important initial skill is to be able to put the informants at their ease and gain their confidence. Essentially this is achieved if the interviewer is genuinely interested in the task, and concerned about learning from the informants. Of equal importance is the practice of customary good manners in greeting, making the necessary introductions and telling the informants the purpose of the interview. This interview may be the first contact of an ongoing relationship, and must therefore also be concluded in a friendly and polite atmosphere. (This, of course, is common courtesy).

It is difficult at the outset to know how long a particular interview is going to take. Sufficient time should be allowed for establishing rapport and for asking all the relevant questions in a relaxed but efficient manner. The interview will probably last no longer than an hour, and more likely 20 to 30 minutes.

Below are some simple hints for interviewing, asking questions and recording answers. Publications providing a more complete description of skills and interview methods, are listed in the annotated bibliography.

3.2.2 Hints for interviewing

1. Always introduce yourself. Give the reason for the interview request. Assure the respondents that the information will be kept confidential.

2. Ask the respondents if they are willing to be interviewed and whether they mind if you take notes, make tape recordings, etc., of the answers.

3. Record the date of interview, names of respondents, and their address, position, age and sex. This is important, both for analysing data and for keeping in contact with informants.

4. Start the interview with the least controversial questions, in order to put informants at their ease and create confidence.

5. During the interview:

    -   encourage responses by not passing judgement on any response, giving advice or commenting in any way;

    -   engage in active listening, repeating answers to make sure you have clearly understood the response;

    -   clarify words and ideas that you have not fully understood and do not assume answers because of your own knowledge and expertise;

    -   inform the respondents when you are going to change the line of questioning so that you can be followed;

    -   know your checklist and which questions are essential;

    -   bring the interview to a close when you think the topic has been exhausted.

6. Always thank respondents for their time, and end an interview by asking if the respondents have any questions for you.

3.2.3 Hints for asking questions

1. Prepare a checklist of general questions, based on the areas identified in the information pyramid, in advance. It is not necessary to prepare separate questions for each category of key informant. The advantages of using the same general questions for all interviews, are that time is saved in preparation and, of more importance, responses are obtained from different sources on the same subject.

2. Keep most questions open-ended, that is questions which encourage respondents to answer in a free-ranging style.

3. Make each question about a single idea, using simple and unambiguous words, and as short as possible. If the initial question is misunderstood it can be clarified.

4. Use "Why" questions sparingly. If used frequently they tend to put informants on the defensive and stop the flow of information.

5. Avoid questions that influence the reply (e.g. "Don't you think that the community nurses should do more home visiting?").

6. Also avoid questions that use negatives (e.g. "Is it not true that ...") thus inviting positive replies.

7. Ask questions in a way that does not reveal the interviewer's bias.

> In posing questions, take into account cultural constraints and find acceptable ways of raising sensitive subjects that are not usually discussed in an open manner.

3.2.4 Individual or group interviews

Both individual and group interviews are undertaken in RPA. Individual interviews are conducted with members of the team and one key informant. They follow the lines of a semi-structured interview as described above.

Individual interviews have the advantage of allowing in-depth probing of various topics without interruptions. It is fairly easy to clarify questions and answers by repeating and/or rephrasing information. The line of questioning is fairly easy to control. In addition, each member of the team of interviewers can have an opportunity to interact with the respondent, allowing information to emerge in a field with which the interviewer is familiar.

The disadvantages include the problems of getting information if the informant is not comfortable or not talkative. There is little spontaneity of answers, and as a result, new ideas or information which has not been foreseen are less likely to emerge. Also, information which the respondent does not want to reveal is likely to remain hidden.

Group interviews, like individual interviews, are usually semi-structured, and are useful for several reasons. They provide the opportunity for interaction, which generates ideas. They also permit interviewers to observe the relations of different key informants with each other, which can reveal information about social views and attitudes. In addition, it may be politically astute to interview members of organizations first together, then individually. In this way, the formal body does not feel threatened by anything an individual might say.

The most popular type of group interview at present is the focus group discussion, which can be defined as a group discussion that gathers together people from similar backgrounds or experiences to discuss a specific topic of interest to the researcher(26). A focus group usually has 8 - 12 participants. The discussion is guided by a facilitator and a recorder takes careful notes. Focus groups provide a range of opinions and ideas about a topic, but cannot indicate relative frequency, i.e. how many people hold these ideas. A guide to focus group interviews by Dawson et al., is available (see Annotated bibliography, section 3).

Among the advantages of group interviews are the following: they are able to produce a lot of information quickly; they identify and explore opinions and attitudes; they indicate a range of belief among key informants; they indicate areas for further questioning in individual interviews; and they often make people feel more comfortable as this is the most common way of communicating among community groups.

They also have several disadvantages: that the team has less control over answers than in individual interviews; the results are often harder to analyse because of the particular social environment, thus care must be taken not to use comments out of context; and they can often be harder to facilitate, particularly by those who have no training in group facilitation. In addition, recording information is more difficult: by hand, because people often talk at the same time and in rapid succession; and/or by tape cassette, because all interviews must be transcribed.

Group interviews, require more careful planning than individual interviews, including the setting of a time, date and place. They may also require permission from the local authority. The team has to be assigned definite roles which are not interchangeable during the interviews. However, in terms of getting a substantial amount of interesting and useful information quickly, they have the potential to overcome the difficulties of preparation and implementation.

These interviewing skills require practice and even for those whose normal work requires different interpersonal skills, a conscious effort must be made to acquire and use these skills.

A word of caution concerning interpretation is necessary. Experience suggests that many teams are tempted to record the number of times an idea is expressed by key informants, and attribute importance to quantifying this information. At this stage of the planning process, it is not the quantity, but the quality of information that is important. That an idea is mentioned a number of times is important, but the exact number of times, or how many key informants mentioned it, has very little relevance.

The number of times that an idea is presented in key informant interviews is only relevant as an indication of the importance of the idea. It gains no more credibility if made into a quantitative measure by recording the number of times it was said, or the number of informants who said it. It is more important in the context of who said it and why.

To answer the question posed by the title for this section, both individual and group interviews are important for RPA as both approaches provide information which is critical for defining problems.

3.2.5 Recording data

It is not necessary to print special forms for the checklist or for recording responses and observations; a notebook can be used for these purposes. On the front cover of the notebook, reminders for the conduct of interviews are recorded, for example:

-   introduce yourself/your group: who you are; why you are here;

-   ask whether the person is willing to be interviewed;

-   ask whether the person is happy for notes to be made on answers;

-   remember to record identification data: name, address, position, age and sex.

The checklist is then written on the first page. In practice, observation and interviewing will often be undertaken together - the one checklist serves as an *aide mémoire* for both purposes. However, when recording, observations should be clearly distinguished from the responses of key informants for easy analysis. This can be achieved by dividing the pages of the notebook into two columns, one for observations and the other for responses.

During the interview, key points should be noted down in the appropriate column of the notebook. No attempt should be made to record everything that is said. The notes can be expanded, if necessary, after the interview, while the content is still fresh in the mind of the interviewer. If verbatim statements are being recorded they must, of course, be written down in full during the interview (or taped and transcribed later). It is also better to make a short note of observations at the time they are made. This note can also be expanded later if necessary. Findings should be written up at the end of each day, while recollections are still fresh. These findings can later be transferred to blank sheets of paper or cards to be placed in the information pyramid.

3.3   Observation skills

As noted in the previous chapter, observations are important both for identifying problems which may not have been discussed with those interviewed, and to confirm or deny information gained through interviews and/or documents.   Several types of observations can be made. The first relates to an examination of the physical environment of the area.   Problems of sanitation, waste disposal, lack of proper roads and poor housing can all be seen during the visits for the interviews. These observations should be recorded and checked against the information given by key informants.

A second type of observation concerns the services provided in the areas of health, housing, education. How well are they managed? Are the records well kept? Are the staff readily available and enthusiastic? Is good supervision being undertaken? Professional experience will be particularly useful in making these observations.

Interviewers might observe whether activities are being carried out to implement legislation regarding services and improvements in the area. Are the benefits to which low-income people are entitled available? Do people accept these benefits? Are the health services promised by primary health care policies available? Are they used?

Finally observations might be made about the attitudes of the key informants during the discussions. Are certain people attempting to manipulate the interview to put across their own view, which may not be representative of wider community views? Do interviewees have "hidden agendas", which they are pursuing in the discussions? What body language do they use?

Observations make good data when undertaken in a systematic and critical way. For this reason, some of the following rules listed in the box are useful.

Some rules for observations

1.   Be sensitive to the situation, and refrain from drawing attention to yourself or making people suspicious of your activities.

2.   Make observations in a way that does not make people feel uncomfortable. For example, you may not be able to take notes because you do not want people to know you are making observations or because you may not have permission to do so. In these cases, you may have to remember what you see, then record later.

3.   Be systematic in your observations. Work towards developing a hypothesis, then test the hypothesis.

4.   Be flexible, and be willing to change your approach in response to the situation.

3.4   Reviewing documents

Documents can provide information to confirm old ideas or develop new ones about community needs. While some documents may be published, most will be unpublished records, for example, vital statistics, clinic records, reports from consultancy groups or foreign donors/nongovernmental organizations. It is important for the team to commit some time and energy in searching out relevant documents, for example, by asking relevant institutions, such as government offices and local universities, whether information is available concerning the area in which the team is working.

It is worth repeating that the "rapid" in rapid participatory appraisal means that the information to be collected is the information that will be used in a quick preliminary assessment of community needs. It is therefore not useful to collect too much information, as time will not be available to analyse it. The professional experience of team members must be used critically in selecting information for the appraisal.

In using records the following hints may be helpful:

1. Reports of surveys by previous investigators may be valuable. A few well organized communities may have prepared reports on issues of major importance. Agencies may have prepared reports for donors or government, or for internal purposes. It is likely that estimates of the infant mortality rate, and perhaps other indicators, will have been made. However, these rates must be interpreted with great caution, as they often represent aggregate data, and therefore hide differences between the better-off people and the poor. Where systematic stratification of information has been undertaken, and disaggregated indicators are available, they provide useful summary information on the health of the population.

2. While records may be poorly maintained, there is likely to be some documentation, such as annual reports, available from the health centres and projects in a community. These should be reviewed with due regard for their likely inaccuracies. There may be official municipal or Ministry of Health reports which refer to the provision of services in the communities being assessed.

3. Legal documents are often difficult to read for those who are not lawyers, while policy documents and health plans are less difficult. The former may be clarified by legal departments within the local authorities. Institutes of social policy or administration may have undertaken reviews of legislation in the light of new policies; these may be helpful.

4. Once relevant data have been identified by scanning the document, they should immediately be recorded in as much detail as is required. The title of the document and other identification details (source, date, author) should be noted with the extract.

3.5   Using projective techniques

In Chapter 1, the importance of visual presentations (pictures or diagrams) for collecting and analysing information in RPAs was highlighted, and one type, an information pyramid, was described (section 1.5). The literature on qualitative methods, shows that information gathering and analysis have greatly benefited from such projective techniques, which also include role play, open-ended stories, and agree and disagree statements. These techniques, adapted from the field of psychology are used to present respondents with stimuli in order to provoke a response or interpretation, overcoming an individual's speaking about topics buried deep in his or her psychological make up. By using a variety of stimuli, these deep-seated feelings can be brought to the surface and expressed.

In qualitative research, the use of such techniques for the purpose of gaining people's reactions to, and views about, a specific topic of interest to the interviewer is becoming more widespread(27). In rapid rural appraisal and participatory rural appraisal, projective techniques that involve visual presentations have made major contributions. One reason, as suggested earlier, is because pictures provide a basis for discussions between professionals and community members; in the past, spoken language alone and the lack of a common background and experience placed almost unsurmountable barriers to gaining valid knowledge. The techniques are particularly useful for gaining information which might not be forthcoming in interviews, and for initiating some important participatory processes which underpin a major objective of the exercise.

Visual presentations can be divided into two categories based on the objectives: pictures for professionals and pictures for partnerships. As the name implies, pictures for professionals are used to create a common understanding among professional members of the team in terms of analytical frameworks, for example, the development of matrices for the purpose of assessing priorities concerning use of resources, problems and/or solutions. In RPA, the use of a feasibility matrix allows the team to assess possible interventions according to criteria set by planners and/or community participants to list a range of options, and then analyse these options in a hierarchy of relationships (section 2.2.7). However, a feasibility matrix could also be used to obtain information from key informants, for example, concerning the food they eat, the health services they use, or the way in which they generate income.

The objective of pictures for partnerships is to create a common framework for a sharing of information between the professionals and the community. Perhaps, mapping exercises are the best known and the most used practice. Community members draw a map which illustrates their perception of a given situation. They can be asked to map their village, indicating the most important institutions such as clinics, schools or religious places. Social mapping encourages local people to identify areas of wealth and poverty. A transect map, drawn on the basis of walking around a specific area and discussing it with community people, presents various points of importance visually. These maps all provide a trigger for discussions among planners and community participants(28). More importantly, they introduce an element of information-sharing, including community members as well as resource holders in the ownership of the information.

There is a wide and continually changing variety of tools and techniques available for both categories. Thies and Grady (see Annotated bibliography, section 5) describe a broad range and give details about how each can be used. Another important source is the Sustainable Agricultural Programme of the International Institute of Environment and Development. Its publication *PLA Notes (formerly entitled RRA Notes)* provides information about a range of experiences using these techniques, and presents innovative adaptations through descriptions of case studies (see Annotated bibliography, section 5).

CHAPTER 4. EXPERIENCE WITH RAPID PARTICIPATORY APPRAISAL

4.1   Project experiences

Since these guidelines were first published in 1988(*14*), they have been used to help make community needs assessments in a range of countries and localities. Because the guidelines were originally developed and field tested in the context of health care for the urban poor, many of these assessments were undertaken in that context. In this section, some of these experiences are reviewed. One example however, examines the use of the guidelines for training health managers in the rural areas of Cameroon, and illustrates a further possibility of their application.

4.1.1 Planning for the urban poor in Bolivia

In 1990, the Bolivian Government decided to develop a PHC project in one of the poor districts in the city of La Paz. The project received support from the Netherlands Government as a part of the Dutch contribution to a larger World Bank programme for upgrading low-income urban areas. In order for the project to reflect the needs and concerns of the local population in the area designated as District Three of the City of El Alto, a needs assessment was undertaken using RPA.

The RPA, based on the original WHO guidelines, was undertaken by a multidisciplinary team responsible to the Ministry of Social Welfare and Public Health. The methods were introduced to the team for three days in April 1991 and the information was collected over the next few weeks. The team met for two days in May 1991 to report findings and define a plan of action. The result of this appraisal became the basis of the plan of operation for the PHC project.

The RPA team worked in groups in nine subdistricts using key informant interviews, observations and documents as the basis for the assessment. The results were published in a document issued by the local municipal health directorate. The framework enabled planners to involve local residents and to discover community needs and priorities. It injected a community participation dimension into a multi- million dollar infrastructure project. Many of those involved in the planning and execution of the entire programme, including officials in the Dutch Government, believe that the RPA approach gave credibility to the project in the context of PHC(*29*).

4.1.2 Training rural health managers in Cameroon

With the support of <u>Deutsche Gesellschaft für Technische Zuammenarbeit</u> [German Technical Development Agency] and in cooperation with the Ministry of Health and the Ministry of Community Development of Cameroon, a five-week participatory training workshop, based on the original WHO guidelines, was conducted(*30*). The purpose of the training was fourfold: to collect information about how health workers and health staff view each other's problems and needs; to identify the communication weakness of health staff at the local level; to improve the skills of health workers to deliver health care in the context of PHC; and to train health workers and supervisors to improve communications for PHC.

The appraisal team consisted of two expatriate facilitators and six local counterparts. The workshop was carried out in three stages. The first included a preparatory discussion by all participants in which agreement on the workshop objectives and on the framework for the community study was reached. This period was also used to enable participants to learn skills for interviewing, observation and socioeconomic ranking, with which to collect and analyse information.

In stage two, participants undertook the field work to collect information for the interacting with rural health staff and community key informants. The information was analysed and then fed back to the community during a series of meetings, and to the rural health staff in a separate discussion.

Stage three was a final workshop in which the findings and priorities of the appraisal were discussed with 15 health workers who were not involved in the training. The participants conducted this workshop by themselves using the skills and methods they had learned and practised with the expatriate facilitators. As a result of this process, there were health workers trained to undertake participatory assessments for each province in the country.

4.1.3 Rapid appraisal for health service restructuring in the South Sefton Health Authority, Merseyside, England

In the summer of 1989, the South Sefton Health Authority in Merseyside, England, decentralized its community based services and created four distinct localities. The existing data were insufficient as a basis for plans for the restructuring, and it was decided to obtain additional information using a method that involved the community in defining its own health needs and formulating action plans(15). The original WHO guidelines were used in undertaking this rapid appraisal.

A team consisting of members of the Health Authority, other municipal agencies including the Housing Authority and Social Services and university researchers came together to undertake the exercise. A two-day workshop was convened at which existing documents were analysed and gaps in information determined. A protocol was designed to set out the specific purpose of the assessment and to identify key informants. The team was then divided into three groups, each containing members from various agencies to provide multisectoral experience.

These groups carried out the field work over a period of 8 weeks, often after normal office hours. At the end of this period, a meeting was convened for one day to analyse the data collected, define problems and set priorities for action. After this meeting a short paper was written and distributed to all those who had participated in the assessment and to the Locality Manager of the health care services in the area. As a result, health managers began to take more of a facilitating role, supporting various actions which the communities decided to undertake themselves. The Locality Manager set up mechanisms for meeting community people to help carry out the actions. Liaison between health, social services, housing and voluntary organizations was strengthened at both the field and managerial levels. The contacts between the team and the community were to continue but on a more infrequent basis through meetings where progress was to be assessed.

4.1.4 Assessing low-income health needs in a general practice in Edinburgh, Scotland

On the basis of the experience of the South Sefton Health Authority described in section 4.1.3, a group of doctors in general practice in a poor area of Edinburgh, Scotland, decided to use the RPA approach to improve the relevance of their care(16). Part of the attraction of a community-needs assessment reflected recent changes in the United Kingdom National Health Service; funding has been decentralized to local practices which are now responsible for allocating these resources. The practice group in Edinburgh, serving a vulnerable community, wished to ensure that its scarce resources were used to the best effect.

The appraisal team consisted of a general practitioner from the practice health centre, the health visitor, the local community education worker, and two local social workers. The team could not work full time on the appraisal, so it was undertaken over three months with each team member contributing four hours a week.

Using the original WHO guidelines, the team devised an interview schedule and pilot-tested the protocol. Interviews were conducted with key informants who included local health service professionals, teachers, workers in voluntary social service organizations and 17 residents selected to represent various age groups, social situations and health problems in the community.

After analysing the results, the team called a meeting to present the findings to all informants, after which two focus groups were conducted to consider priorities and explore possible interventions. Informants also made suggestions for improvements in general practice health service delivery. A final report was circulated by the team, and a local newspaper published the detailed findings and invited comments.

The findings pointed to a number of corrective measures that could be undertaken immediately and easily by the general practice. These were implemented. In addition, the appraisal indicated community concerns that had no direct links with health service delivery; demands for an improvement in bus services met with a positive response from the appropriate authority.

The team was pleased with the flexibility of then RPA approach to planning which enables solutions to be found at the time problems are identified.

4.2   Benefits and limitations of rapid participatory appraisal

Experiences have suggested that RPA has a number of benefits for planners seeking community responsive and sustainable programmes, including the following:

- RPA is relatively cheap to conduct because limited time and expenditure are required for data collection. The use of professionals to make up the appraisal team might seem to be a large expenditure of resources. However, because of their experience and role in allocating resources, their use is cost-effective.

- RPA uses community knowledge. It relies on the views and knowledge of local residents, and therefore taps resources that are easily available, and can provide in-depth information about the area. Further, the involvement of community members in problem identification helps to build a mutual credibility between health service delivery personnel and health service beneficiaries, which is critical for mobilizing scarce resources to meet the health needs of the most vulnerable people.

- RPA involves resource holders and can be managed by the planning team. It allows the managers of a programme to participate in identifying the problems. Planners have found that RPA has alerted them to community problems previously unknown to them. It has also allowed them to establish working relationships with community members that ensure community input to some mutually identified solutions and health interventions.

However, for RPA to be useful in planning to improve health among the poor, it is important to understand its limitations. As has been emphasized previously, RPA is a critical step in the planning process for a plan of action based on community perceived needs.

- RPA is **not** a detailed household survey which quantifies the size of the problem. Once problems have been identified and given priorities by planners and key informants, a small household survey may be necessary (see section 2.3.1). However, this is not the same as an RPA.

- RPA is **not** a collection of interviews based on grass-roots informants. The informants are chosen because they are able to represent the views of a group or groups of people in the community. Further collection of individual community opinions would not only complicate the analysis, but would also lengthen the process.

- RPA is **not** a basis for comparison of problems in different areas in the same district, or in other districts; it is specific to the situation for which planning for health improvements is to be undertaken. Because it is a step in the planning process for a particular group of people, it cannot be seen as an isolated collection of data outside the planning context. It might, however, highlight common problems and provide guidance for actions in other communities, or in other low-income groups in other districts.

Further, it is important to note the ever present problem of bias in the information collected. Information can be biased by inaccuracy because, for example, team members fail to carefully record information, to acknowledge limitations of the data collection and/or fail to cross-check information. Bias can be a result of poor representation, where key informants are chosen from groups that share similar views about a problem, if not offset by informants from a different background who might have a different view (e.g. interviewing only informants who are officials and omitting those who have no official post). Bias might also come from cultural inappropriateness, where interviews do not use acceptable means that allow valid answers (e.g. using questionnaires among semi-literates). Bias might result from the interviewer's own subjectivity, where what is heard is what the interviewer wants to hear, or data may be manipulated to support a view held, possibly for emotional reasons, by a team member. However, bias can be overcome - when the sources described above are recognized, it is possible to take corrective action. Team members have the collective responsibility to see that everything possible is done to overcome any possible distortion of information or interpretation of data.

4.3   Contributions to community health development

The above descriptions of the use of RPA, both in the field and in training, has highlighted a number of contributions to the area of health development. In the PHC context, the RPA approach has helped to translate some RPA principles into concrete experiences. For example, the principle of equity has been realized by focusing the assessment on low-income communities, so that the more disadvantaged people are provided with opportunities to participate both in data collection, and in decisions about resource allocation based on this information. An important extension of this process is the potential to empower these members of the community through ownership of the information.

The principle of participation shapes the RPA approach - RPA was expressly designed to enable beneficiaries to be involved in needs assessment.

The principle of multisectoral cooperation is respected by using multidisciplinary teams of people employed in different social sectors and with programme responsibility and accountability, who bring to the exercise a range of professional skills and experiences. This breadth has enabled RPA teams to process information quickly, by focusing on the critical aspects of problems, and by using experts to assess and apply the information collected.

Two further contributions, outside the PHC framework, can be identified. First, RPA has developed credible ways of applying both qualitative and quantitative methods for assessment. The by-product has been an enriched body of information which reflects both the perception and magnitude of community health problems.

Secondly, RPA has provided programme managers with the tools and experience with which to collect, analyse and apply community information using their own skills and efforts. Too often in the past, information was collected by those whose rigid training in survey techniques did not admit a broader, more comprehensive approach. With survey tools in the hands of managers, assessments can be rapidly completed and acted upon. In addition, managers have personal contacts with the groups whose needs are being assessed. Promoting these contacts, and involving community people in programme decisions and implementation, should enhance both the continuity and the sustainability of the programmes.

REFERENCES

1.   *Primary health care. Report of the International Conference on Primary Health Care, Alma-Ata*, 1978. Geneva, World Health Organization, 1978.

2.   Institute of Development Studies (1981). *"Rapid rural appraisal, special issue"*, IDS Bulletin, 12: 4.

3.   Chambers R. (1983). *Rural Development: Putting the Last First*, London: Longman.

4.   Mascarenhas J, et al. (1991). *"Participatory Rapid Appraisal: Proceedings of the February 1991 Bangalore PRA Trainers Workshop"*, RRA Notes, 13.

5.   Chambers R. (1994). "The origins and practice of participatory rural appraisal". *World Development*, **22**(7): 953-969

6.   Chambers R. (1981). "Rapid rural appraisal: rationale and repertoire" *Public Administration and Development*, **1**: 95-106.

7.   Selwyn BJ, et al. (1989). "Rapid Epidemiologic Assessment: The evolution of a new discipline-introduction", *International Journal of Epidemiology*, 18.

8.   Scrimshaw S, Hurtado E. (1988). *Rapid Assessment Procedures for Nutrition and Primary Health Care*, Tokyo, The United Nations University, UNICEF, Los Angeles: UCLA Latin American Centre Publications, 1988.

9.   Bentley M, et al. (1988). "Rapid ethnographic assessment: applications in diarrhoea management in Nigeria and Peru", *Social Science and Medicine*, **27**(l), 107-16.

10. Pelto G. (1992). *"Developing a focused ethnographic study for the WHO Acute Respiratory Infection (ARI) Control programme"*. In: Scrimshaw, N.S. and Gleason, G.R. eds, RAP: Rapid Assessment Procedures, Boston: International Nutrition Foundation for Developing Countries.

11. Kashyap P, Young R. (1989). *Rapid Assessment of Community Nutrition Problems*, Ottawa, IDRC.

12. Varkevisser C, et al. (1993). *Rapid appraisal of health and nutrition in a PHC project in Pahou, Benin*, Amsterdam, Royal Tropical Institute, and Cotonou: Centre Régional pour le Développement et la Santé.

13. Rifkin SB, Annett H. (1991). "Using rapid appraisal for data collection in poor urban areas". In: Yesudian, C.A.K. ed. *Primary Health Care*, Bombay: Tata Institute of Social Sciences.

14. World Health Organization. *Guidelines for rapid appraisal to assess community needs*, Geneva: WHO/SHS/NHP/88.4, 1988.

15. Ong, Bie Nio Ong et al. (991). "Rapid Appraisal in an Urban setting, an example from the Developed World. *Social Science and Medicine*, **32**(8).

16. Murray SA, et al. (1994). "Listening to local voices: adapting rapid appraisal to health and social needs in general practice", *British Medical Journal*, **308**: 12.

17. Banerji D. *Social Sciences and Health Service Development in India: Sociology of Formation of an Alternative Paradigm*, New Delhi, Lok Paksh, 1986.

18. Harpham T, et al. (eds) (1988). *In the Shadow of the City: Community Health and the Urban Poor*, Oxford, Oxford University Press.

19. Levine A. (1984). "A model for health projections using knowledgeable informants", *World Health Statistics Quarterly*, **37**: 306-313.

20. Morerea RG, Levine A, Ray DK, (1980). "Crash" health manpower planning: a method for developing countries", *World Health Forum*, **1**(2): 34-44.

21. Conway G, McCraken J, Pretty J. (1987). *Training Notes for Agro-ecosystem analysis and Rapid Rural Appraisal*, London: International Institute for Environment and Development.

22. *ZOPP An Introduction to the Method*. Deutsche Gesellschaft für Technische Zuammenarbeit, Eschborn. March, 1987.

23. Hill AG, David PH. (1988). "Monitoring changes in child mortality: new methods for use in developing countries. "*Health Policy and Planning*", **3**(3): 214-226: Oxford University Press.

24. United Nations ACC Task Force on Rural Development, Panel on Monitoring and Evaluation. *Monitoring and Evaluation: Guiding Principles*, Rome, IFAD Publications, 1985.

25. Feuerstein MT. (1986). *Partners in Evaluation: Evaluating Development and Community Programmes with Participants*, London, Macmillan.

26. Dawson S, et al. (1993). *A Manual for the Use of Focus Groups*, Boston, International Nutrition Foundation for Developing Countries.

27. Maier B, Gorgen R, Kielmann AA, Diesfeld HJ, Korte R. (1994). *Assessment of the District Health System Using Qualitative Methods*, London: Deutsche Gesellschaft für Technische Zuammernarbeit (GTZ), Institut für Tropenhygiene und Öffenliches Gesundheitswesn, Macmillan.

28. Chambers R. (1992). *Rural Appraisal: rapid, relaxed and participatory*, Brighton, Institute of Development Studies, (IDS Discussion Paper 311).

29. Proyecto de Foralecimiento de la Atencion Primaria en el Distrito III de la Cuidad de El Alto, La Paz, Bolivia, *Diagnostico Rapido Situacion de la Salud en El Distrito III, El Alto, La Paz*: Directora Unidad Sanitaria El Alto, 1991.

30. de Koning K, Bichmann W. (1993). "Listening to communities and health workers", *Learning for Health*, 3.

ANNOTATED BIBLIOGRAPHY

The publications listed below provide details of the methods, skills and techniques used in carrying out a rapid participatory appraisal. They have been selected because they are easily available and, for the most part, fairly inexpensive. It is hoped that this list will provide readers with the information necessary to put into practice the approaches described in the guidelines.

1. Epidemiology

Beaglehole R, Bonita R, Kjellström T. *Basic epidemiology*, Geneva, World Health Organization, 1993 (IBSN 92 4154446 5).

This publication describes how to carry out epidemiological studies. It is a clear and useful "how to" manual. The early chapters define epidemiology and discuss ways of measuring health and disease. Subsequent chapters focus on a review of the types of epidemiological studies, basic statistics, causation in epidemiology and epidemiology and prevention. There are specific chapters dealing with epidemiology and public health, which include the role of epidemiology in communicable diseases, clinical care, and environmental and occupational health problems, and a discussion about the application of epidemiology in health systems and health policy. The final chapter describes how epidemiological knowledge and skills can be developed further and includes information on setting up a research project, critical reading of published reports on projects, and further reading and training.

Coggon D, Rose G, Barker DJP. *Epidemiology for the uninitiated*, London, British Medical Journal Publishing Group, 1993 (ISBN 0 7279 0770 0).

This book provides a good clear introduction to basic epidemiological concepts and terminology. It is useful for those who have little or no knowledge of the subject.

Vaughan JP, Morrow RH, eds. *Manual of epidemiology for district health management*, Geneva, World Health Organization, 1989 (ISBN 92 4 154404).

This manual provides clear and simple instructions for applying epidemiological techniques to obtain information for district health management. It gives details of how to set up an information system, surveillance of diseases, controlling an epidemic, conducting surveys, establishing record forms and coding, data processing and analysis, and presenting and communicating information. The final chapter provides a glossary of definitions. This manual is particularly appropriate for those working in developing countries.

2.   Survey methods and techniques

Kielmann AA, Janovsky K, Annett H. *Assessing district health needs, services and systems*, London, African Medical Research Foundation and Macmillan, 1991 (ISBN 0 333 53885 4).

This is a manual designed for national health planners, district team members, technical advisers to ministries of health, and staff of training and research institutes to enable them to collect information for making an assessment of needs and problems in the community in a rapid manner. With a criterion of obtaining the minimum information necessary to begin programmes, the manual is divided into three parts. The first part gives an overview of the succeeding survey protocols, and gives some guidance on which to choose in order to achieve the objectives of the assessment. The second part provides protocol examples for: background information of the area under survey; district health management and support systems; primary health care facility information; rural and/or district hospital information; community participation and traditional medical systems; patterns of mortality; and community and household information. Each module explains how to implement the survey and suggests how to analyse the information and interpret the results. The third part makes suggestions about how to summarize the analysis and present a report. The protocols give examples of the types of questions that are important in a rapid assessment, and the areas that are critical for planning.

Lutz W, Chalmers J, Hepburn W, Lockerbie L. *Health and community surveys*, Vol.1 & 2, London and Basingstoke, Macmillan, International Epidemiological Association and World Health Organization, 1992 (Vol. 1, ISBN 0 333 57449 4; Vol. 2, ISBN 0 333 57450 8).

These two volumes, written in dialogue form, take the reader through the steps for organizing surveys to investigate health problems. The first volume focuses on the planning and organizing of a survey, using available information and selecting the survey sample. The second volume describes questionnaire design, methods of interviewing and recording information and presentation of the results. It is a clear step-by-step presentation, describing the uses and the limitations of each method.

Pratt B, Loizos P. *Choosing research methods*, Oxford, Oxfam, 1992 (ISBN 0 85598 177 6).

Although set in the context of information for development workers, this concise book gives guidance for developing research which is action linked, focusing a specific intervention in any context. It provides practical advice on the ways in which to design the information collection, and on the methods available for collecting the data. It starts by examining issues concerning research design, including the level of participation by the group to be studied, and the expectations that may be present. The second chapter investigates planning the research, including the amount of time, the unit of analysis, the questions of scientific soundness and choice of the researchers. Next, a range of methods, including rapid appraisal are described. General issues of appropriate indicators and validation are also discussed. A check list of questions is provided, and additional information is given on questionnaire design, some "high-tech", high-cost research methods, logical framework analysis, women and evaluation, and methods and approaches to action research programmes.

3.   Qualitative research

Dawson S, Manderson L, Tallo V. *A manual for the use of focus groups*, Boston, International Nutrition Foundation for Developing Countries, 1993 ISBN 0 9635522 2 8).

This publication is designed to help those involved in disease control programmes to learn more about the social and cultural issues relating to disease transmission, control and prevention. The first part describes training in the focus group method for the team leader, and considers the reasons for choosing this method, how to design the study, how to select and train staff, how to select participants in a focus group, how to develop the line of questioning, how to manage the information collected, and how to analyse the results. Part two describes staff training for focus group discussions, and gives details on how to facilitate such discussions and analyse the information obtained.

Maier B, Gorgen R, Kielmann AA, Diesfeld HJ, Korte R. *Assessment of the district health system using qualitative methods*, London, Deutsche Gesellschaft für Technische Zuammernarbeit (GTZ), Institut für Tropenhygiene und Öffentliches Gesundheitswesen, Macmillan, 1994 (ISBN 0 333 59786 9).

This slim volume describes the use of qualitative methods for gaining information about health beliefs and behaviours, using examples from developing countries. The reasons for using qualitative techniques for information for planning at the district level are outlined and a range of techniques described, each illustrated by its use in a specific situation. The techniques include interviews, observation, interactive and/or projective techniques, and techniques for data recording and analysis. A list of health-related questions in which qualitative methods would be appropriate to research is also provided. The book has a bibliography to direct the reader to information about the how to use the techniques, and situations to which they might be appropriately applied.

Patton MQ. *Qualitative evaluation and research methods*, London, Sage Publications, 1990 (ISBN 0 8039 3779 2)

This publication is one of the better texts on applied qualitative research. Clearly written and with numerous examples, the author describes, from first-hand experience, the translation of theory into practice, using qualitative methods for programme evaluation.

The first part reviews in some depth the conceptual basis for qualitative inquiry, including the nature of this type of inquiry, strategic themes, theoretical orientations and particularly appropriate applications. Part two details the designing of qualitative studies, field work strategies, and observation and interviewing methods. Part three examines analysis and interpretation, and ways in which to increase both the quality and credibility of this type of research. There is an extensive bibliography.

Taylor SJ, Bogdan R. *Introduction to qualitative research methods*, New York, John Wiley & Sons, 1984 (ISBN 0 47 88947 4).

This volume is designed to assist those who wish to undertake qualitative research. The introduction discusses qualitative methods in general, and the conceptual tradition underlying their use. The first part explains how to collect data, including participant observation, in-depth interviewing, and some more creative data collection techniques. It also describes data analysis. Part two describes how to write up the findings, and how these findings can and cannot influence programmes and policy. Although examples are drawn from the United States of America, the book is valuable because it gives details of how to use the methods, and records experiences in application of data to health programmes and policy.

Qualitative research for health programmes, Geneva, World Health Organization (unpublished document, WHO/MHN/PSF/94.3).

This manual, shortly to be published, can be obtained by writing to the Division of Mental Health, World Health Organization, 1211 Geneva 27, Switzerland. It is a clear guide to using qualitative research in investigating health problems. After an introduction, which examines the use of qualitative research and its relation to quantitative research, the document describes how to use a number of techniques specifically within the context of obtaining information about health beliefs and practices. It then discusses various aspects of sampling techniques and study design. There is a chapter on data analysis and presentation, and one on examples for using qualitative techniques. A glossary of concepts, summary tables of data collection methods, a bibliography of resources and a resource list of computer programmes are also provided.

4.   Communication skills training

Johnston MP, Rifkin SB. *Health care together*, London, Macmillan, 1987 (ISBN 0 333 44348 9).

This book describes 41 exercises which are designed to improve skills in communication, team-work, leadership and community development among health workers. The success of a rapid participatory appraisal depends on clear communication and a good working atmosphere among planners and the beneficiaries. Using these exercises professionals can gain the skills to create this environment. Each exercise is explained in detail, including the objectives, the length of time it takes to complete, the most appropriate situation, the materials required, the activities and discussions involved, and the conclusions to be drawn.

5.   Rapid appraisals

PLA Notes

These notes (formerly entitled *RPA Notes*) are published by the Sustainable Agriculture Programme of the International Institute for Environment and Development. Their object is to allow practitioners of rapid rural appraisal and participating rural appraisal throughout the world to share their field experiences and methodological innovations. The selections have no formal format. There is no copyright on the materials, and recipients are urged to circulate the information for non-profit purposes only. They can be obtained by writing to:

> Sustainable Agricultural Programme
> International Institute for Environment and Development
> 3 Endsleigh Street
> London WC1H ODD, England

Scrimshaw N, Gleason GR, eds. *Rapid assessment procedures*, Boston, International Nutrition Foundation for Developing Countries, 1992 (ISBN 0 9635522 0 1).

This volume is a collection of papers presented at a conference on rapid assessment procedures (RAPs) held in 1990 and supported by WHO and UNICEF. The first section looks at the expanding role of qualitative research in the context of RAPs, using examples for projects in the health and nutrition field. The next section looks at the experiences of RAPs and their continual development using case studies from Africa, Asia and the Americas. Section three describes community participation and rapid rural appraisal as a complement to and a reflection of RAPs examining both the conceptual and practical dimensions. The final sections look at the institutionalization of RAPs, training for RAPs, and the effective use of RAPs for decision-making. The book presents a wide overview of conceptual developments and experiences in using RAPs for needs assessment and evaluation.

Scrimshaw S, Hutardo E. *Rapid assessment procedures*, Toyko, United Nations University, 1988 (ISBN 0 87903 111 5 (U.S.)).

This manual gives detailed instructions for carrying out rapid assessment procedures (RAPs). The first chapter discusses the application of anthropology to health programmes, and the second describes how to apply anthropological methods in undertaking an RAP. The next chapter gives details of focus group techniques. Chapter four discusses selection, training and supervision of field workers. The concluding chapters focus on data analysis and presentation in the final report. Data collection guides, in the form of questions the interviewer should ask, including descriptions of the environment as well as the perceptions of those interviewed, are also provided.

Thies J, Grady H. *Participatory rapid appraisal for community development*, London, International Institute for Environment and Development and Save the Children, 1991 (ISBN 0 905347 97 8).

This is a "how to" manual, which enables the user to use some of the more innovative techniques emerging from rapid rural appraisal and participatory rapid appraisal PRA. Written in the form of a training session, it begins by giving the participants the objectives of a workshop. The idea of PRA is introduced, noting its background, history, relationship with other research methods, its limitations and its place in the project cycle. The next section provides details of how to use a range of tools and techniques to involve local people, in partnership with planners, in obtaining information for the development of projects. Background information and an overview of the exercise is presented, followed by a description about how it should be taught to workshop participants. Each presentation includes materials which can be photocopied and used to support the exercise. The final section discusses putting PRA into practice, and focuses on designing the research, carrying out the field work, analysing and presenting the data, writing the report, preparing an action plan for follow up, and evaluating the training.

Varkevisser CM, Alihonou E, Inoussa S. *Rapid appraisal of health and nutrition in a PHC project in Pahou, Benin*, Amsterdam, Royal Tropical Institute, 1993 (ISBN 90 6832 079 3).

This publication documents the use of rapid appraisal to develop a health and nutrition project in Benin - an example of how the rapid appraisal method, based on the guidelines presented here, can be applied in the field. Details are given of how the team developed the methodology in Pahou and how it was applied in conjunction with a longer quantitative survey. The results of the work are presented and recommendations are made. The final section assesses the methodology and its use in this type of project.

ANNEX I

TIMETABLE FOR THE 10-DAY RAPID APPRAISAL PROCESS

1. Preparation

- Contact facilitator. It may be necessary to do this a least two months before the date of the workshop, to ensure that the facilitator is available when required.

- Select and contact participants at least one month before the workshop.

- Arrange venue for the workshop. Probably several weeks in advance.

Do not forget to prepare a budget and arrange funds for holding the workshop and for the rapid appraisal as a whole.

---

2. Workshop outline

Day 1

Introduction	3 hours
- introduce workshop and participants	
- review urban health problems	
Presentation by the facilitator outlining the purpose and methodology of rapid appraisal	5 hours

Day 2

Use of the information pyramid to develop a checklist for data collection	8 hours

Day 3

Selection of data sources (documents, key informants, observations)	2 hours
Preparation of a plan of action for data collection	1 hour
Exercises to practise skills in semi-structured interviewing	5 hours

Day 4

Document scan		4 hours
Field interviews		4 hours

Day 5

Field interviews (continued)		8 hours

Day 6

Field interviews (continued)		4 hours
Data analysis to sort the data collected and agree on the major health problems		4 hours

Day 7

Data analysis (continued)		4 hours
Field interviews to determine community priorities regarding the problems previously identified		4 hours

Day 8

Finalization of analysis and report of findings		4 hours
Definition of priorities		4 hours

Day 9

Definition of priorities (continued)		4 hours
Preparation of plan of action		4 hours

Day 10

Finalization of draft workshop report and preparation for presentation of report to community leaders and municipal authorities		4 hours
Presentation of report		2 hours
Revision of workshop report in light of feedback from the presentation		2 hours

------

ANNEX II

TIMETABLE FOR THE EXTENDED RAPID APPRAISAL PROCESS

1. Preparation
See Annex I

2. Outline of introductory workshop

Day 1

Introduction	3 hours
- introduce workshop and participants	
- review urban health problems	
Presentation by the facilitator outlining the purpose and methodology of rapid appraisal	5 hours

Day 2

Use of the information pyramid to develop a checklist for data collection	8 hours

Day 3

Selection of data sources (documents, key informants, observations)	2 hours
Preparation of a plan of action for data collection	1 hour
Exercises to practise skills in semi-structured interviewing	5 hours

3. Data collection

Implementation of the plan of action agreed in the introductory workshop	several weeks

4. Outline of final workshop

Day 1

Finalization of analysis and report of findings	4 hours
Definition of priorities	4 hours

Day 2

Definition of priorities (continued)	4 hours
Preparation of plan of action	4 hours

ANNEX III

DATA FOR INFORMATION PYRAMIDS

The basis for collecting and analysing data in rapid participatory appraisals (RPAs) to assess community health needs is the information pyramid: the base level of the pyramid contains information about community structures, interests and capacity to act; the next level has information about the environmental, socioeconomic and disease and disability features; the third level covers the provision, accessibility and acceptability of health, environmental and social services; and the final level concentrates on government policies. Planning must be built on a strong community base. The sections below indicate areas about which information may be usefully collected and the reasons why this information might be useful.

It is not necessary or useful to collect information about each topic, but it is important to be aware that each topic might provide information to help you make a good plan of action. It is the quality not the quantity of information that is important.

1. Building the base: information about communities

The descriptions given here of information at the community level are less detailed than those of information on the environment and service provision in sections 2 and 3, despite the fact that more information is needed. This apparent contradiction is because relevant data about communities depend on the situation in each specific community, and are not so easily divided into defined categories. Much of the information will be collected through discussions and observations, and will provide a general assessment of community structures and capacities, rather than specific data about one area. It is the general description, and the analysis based on this description, that forms the base of the information pyramid.

1.1 Community composition

Identify the major groups in the area and define their common interests.

Many low-income communities are composed of different linguistic, tribal and/or cultural groups, often sharing only a common geographical area and a struggle for scarce resources. For the information pyramid, it is important to define the groups that compose the community, to see which groups share interests, which groups are dominant and which have least access to the few resources, and understand why this may be so. Competition among groups should also be noted, and the leaders of various subgroups should be identified.

1.2 Community organization and structures

Describe the structure of the community and the types of organization found, and determine whose interests the organizations represent.

People living in the same geographical area develop structures and organizations that define the relations they have with one another. Community structure is built on various groupings, according to social class, caste, level of education, type of employment, and income level, etc. These groups come together formally in organizations to develop and support activities, which may be supported by the national government, or locally where strong families or alliances form to exercise some control over life in the community. They include national political party organizations, women's organizations, voluntary and non-governmental organizations and charities like International Rotary. Organizations and structures can either help or impede the introduction of new ideas and activities in a community. They can also facilitate or obstruct assistance and support given to more marginalized people.

1.3 Community capacities

Assess the capacity of the community to mobilize, organize and support a common set of activities.

Community capacity to take action on problems that affect the lives of its members depends on the strength of existing organizations, the role of community people in managing community-based programmes, their participation in defining priorities for community programmes, and their ability and willingness to contribute personal resources to community activities. Understanding community composition, interests and structures, and the types and strengths of community organizations, will help in determining the capacity of the community to take action for health improvements. As the success of programmes depends on this capacity, the more it is taken into account, the greater the chance that plans will achieve their objectives.

2. Describing the environment and the disease blocks

At the second level of the information pyramid, the concern is to develop a profile of those aspects of the community's environment that have major implications for health. Of greatest importance are:

- the physical environment, in particular, housing, water, sanitation, solid waste disposal and the main physical features of the location;

- the socioeconomic environment, in particular, job opportunities in the formal sector, earnings in the informal sector, and cultural/historical traditions that promote or hinder good health;

- disease and disability, in particular, the prevalence of malnutrition, communicable diseases, trauma, high fertility, maternal mortality, physical and mental handicap, and chronic problems due to pollution and stress.

2.1 The physical environment

Describe the quality and availability of housing.

The adequacy of provision of housing can be assessed by the numbers of individuals or families sharing a room and/or the type of material used for the construction of dwellings.

It is important to clarify the legal status of residents in tenements and settlements, as this influences residents' motivation and ability to work for improvements in their living conditions. People may:

- have full legal ownership of their dwelling;
- hold possession "rights";
- rent their property, under a variety of arrangements from a range of owners.

However, settlements may have no legal existence, and therefore be excluded from entitlement to municipal services or protection from summary dissolution. Such circumstances can create a sense of insecurity, powerlessness and hopelessness in a community, and expose it to exploitation by unscrupulous persons. There may also be a substantial number of "residents" of settlements who have no house and live in the open.

The range in the physical structure of houses should be noted. The adequacy of physical structure in relation to prevailing climatic conditions should also be assessed. In urban settlements, for example, the most recent and least substantial homes are likely to have the fewest amenities, though they may be less crowded than long established down-town tenements.

Investigate access to a sufficient water supply of reasonable quality.

The water available should be sufficient for drinking, bathing, food preparation and domestic hygiene. Where the sewage disposal system is dependent on water, a large flow will be essential to keep the system operational. Sufficient water of reasonable quality for drinking is particularly important. In rural areas, there may be considerable seasonal variation in access to water; even during the wet season women and children may have to walk long distances to collect reasonably safe water. In urban settings, a piped system may have low pressure and intermittent supply; its accessibility is determined by whether it is connected to each house or individual dwelling within buildings, or to a community tap. A majority of households may rely upon purchasing water from a vendor, and the price may be exorbitant. Some may rely on rain water, others on waste water.

Where a piped system exists it may be inadequate for a variety of reasons, including absolute scarcity in relation to the numbers to be served, preferential supply to privileged sections of the city, illegal connections to the system; the latter can also lead to contamination of the water and wastage through leakage. Where the public water system is inadequate, the community may lack the motivation to maintain it.

Examine methods of excreta disposal indicating the prevalence of each. Note any plans by the local authority, landlords, or community effort, to introduce improved methods. Are the plans likely to be implemented and how soon?

Common methods for disposal of human excreta are: wet and dry pit latrines, overhung latrines, "wrap and carry" defecation trenching grounds, and defecation in open drains; all of these methods are inadequate. In long established, inner city tenements, or in settlements where improvements have been undertaken, water-carried sewage systems may exist, either in individual houses or for communal use.

Assess the adequacy of the means for solid waste disposal.

Solid waste is often a fire hazard. Its accumulation can block drainage channels, and thereby help create standing water and breeding-sites for disease vectors and rodents. Communities may be totally lacking in efforts at solid waste management, with indiscriminate disposal of refuse by residents, and non-existent services. Alternatively community practices may serve to minimize the accumulation of solid waste, and this can be complemented by some service provision.

Examine the level of standing water in the community.

Standing water is a hazard as a breeding-site for disease vectors and, if substantial, to very young children; it also has considerable nuisance value for residents. It can arise from a total lack of drainage or from drains blocked by general rubbish or "converted" to sewers. A determinant of water stagnation is the geographical location of a settlement.

Does the geographical location of a settlement create health hazards?

The situation of settlements may predispose them to flooding from nearby rivers, or from monsoon rains. Those built up hillsides may be liable to landslides, particularly during the wet season. In cities, extensive rubbish dumps, which often accommodate settlements and which may be a source of income, also contain hazards ranging from broken bottles to considerable accumulations of toxic waste from industry.

Factories producing heavy industrial and toxic items without adequate safeguards are hazardous to health, both as regards general environmental pollution and the risk of industrial accidents. Identification of these risks is important and it may be possible to render the factories safer; the community may value the proximity of the opportunities for work without the expense of travel.

2.2 The socioeconomic environment

2.2.1 Education

Assess the general level of education and describe opportunities for further education.

The levels of literacy and the opportunities for literacy that exist in a community are significant for the creation and maintenance of self-reliance and hygiene standards. In relation to the care of young children, female literacy is most important. However, good standards of adult literacy in general improve a community's organizational capacity, and provide the possibility of access to a wider range of jobs.

2.2.2 Economy

Explore the means of cash income.

In rural areas, food is still obtained almost directly from the land. This means that a cash income is not always necessary to get enough to eat.

In contrast, the physical survival of urban dwellers depends on a cash income; the adequacy of that income will be a major determinant of the quality of life. The means by which cash is obtained will also have important repercussions on the health and social welfare of individuals, and their communities.

The employment opportunities available for both men and women are limited by a number of constraints. The absolute availability of work in the city is the major constraint. Available work may not be accessible for a variety of reasons: the cost of transport, inadequate levels of education, insufficient appropriate skills. Exploitative child labour has serious effects on the health and development of the children, while excluding adults, who are more expensive to employ, from work opportunities.

A frequent source of cash is the re-processing of the discarded surplus of industry and the privileged classes. To obtain sufficient cash for a family to live on most members of the family will be involved in scavenging and processing "waste" during daylight hours. Shoe-cleaning, car "watching", and a host of similar informal jobs may be a means of obtaining cash for a significant number of individuals and family units.

For many, the only means of earning cash for food is through engaging in illegal activities, which may or may not be detrimental to society as a whole. Examples include begging, prostitution, and involvement in illicit drug networks.
Others may turn to stealing.

2.2.3 Child welfare

Try to gain a sense of child welfare.

In rural communities, children may, from an early age, spend much of their time in household work and work on the land. Girls in particular may be denied access to education because of the value of their labour in the family. Children may be separated from their parents in order to work and care for elderly relatives. Children in urban settlements may be at particular risk because they live in extreme poverty in close proximity to affluence. In addition to exploitative child labour, the sexual exploitation of children, both male and female, for financial gain may be widespread in cities. General child abuse may also be a significant and increasing problem, particularly in many urban situations. A conspiracy of silence may cover these matters, but they must be uncovered and addressed.

2.3 Disease and disability

Identify the major disease problems in the community and describe the causes of these problems.

While clinic records may give some evidence of these problems, they are often a questionable source of information since they may be inaccurate, or they may not indicate the areas people come from. Furthermore, they reveal nothing about people who seek care in other places, or cannot afford to seek care at all.

Below are some of the diseases about which information might be sought. Observations and interviews should provide data which, when combined with discussions with health staff and an examination of clinic records, will present a picture of disease problems in the community.

2.3.1 Malnutrition

Malnutrition is not only a major childhood disease in its own right, but also a co-factor in other diseases, particularly infectious diseases. Identification of malnutrition as a problem and a crude assessment of its prevalence are of particular importance, as it may not have been recognized by the community, or accorded a high place in their list of problems. Night blindness, due to vitamin A deficiency, and anaemia may be particular nutrition-related problems where practical intervention is feasible. Among the most deprived parts of a community, severe degrees of general childhood malnutrition may be common.

2.3.2 Communicable diseases

These largely preventable diseases remain the major immediate causes of morbidity and mortality, particularly among children. Acute respiratory infections and diarrhoeal diseases are probably the most important disease complexes and are particularly hazardous to young children, especially those who are malnourished. Measles epidemics of large magnitude are likely in overcrowded housing conditions. The deformities poliomyelitis can cause are a particular handicap in the marginal existence of urban slums. Tuberculosis is a major and often increasing cause of morbidity and premature death. Sexually transmitted diseases, which also infect children, may be common; with the acquired immune deficiency syndrome (AIDS) a particularly lethal hazard. Malaria may not officially "exist" in a city, and yet be a common disease for some urban inhabitants as well as those in rural areas.

2.3.3 Trauma

Road traffic accidents are an increasingly significant cause of trauma in rural areas, complementing the traditional causes of accidents: unsafe agricultural practices and inadequate protection from cooking fires in the home. The physical and social conditions of the urban environment increase the risks of suffering physical trauma and diseases associated with stress. The prevalence of accidents among children and young adults in particular, in the home, at work and on the road, may be a cause of significant concern in a community. Trauma from violence, perhaps related to crime, may also be a concern.

In settlements more recently formed or those with particularly mobile populations, anxiety and other disturbed mental states may be a significant but unrecognized burden for many. In longer-established settlements and among the more wealthy members of urban communities, cardiovascular disease can be an important cause of ill health, particularly affecting middle-aged men responsible for earning cash for family survival.

2.3.4 Womens' health

In many rural communities, women carry out a disproportionate amount of the total work; not only are they solely responsible for work in the home, they are often also responsible for physically demanding work on the land, collecting water, and gathering fuel. This burden is detrimental to their health, especially if cultural and social customs do not provide for extra rest and better food during pregnancy and lactation. In a relatively high percentage of urban families, a woman, often a single parent, may have prime or sole responsibility for the family's survival and well-being. Many women spend long hours in low-paid employment, in addition to their work in the home; they may be undernourished and exposed to the risk of sexually transmitted disease and/or frequent pregnancies, with problems of illegal abortion and poor care at childbirth. Their particular concerns and needs should be addressed, not just for their benefit, but because their health will largely determine their capacity to care for the children.

2.3.5 Chronic and degenerative diseases

The elderly urban population is increasing rapidly, and is vulnerable to diseases that are likely to go unrecognized. In urban communities, elderly people have to be much more self-sufficient than is usual in traditional rural environments. But the characteristic diseases to which they are prone, for example, heart disease, stroke, diabetes, arthritis and senile dementia, reduce their mobility and capacity to provide for themselves. The worst effects of some of these diseases, such as high blood pressure leading to stroke, and diabetes leading to gangrene and amputations, could be prevented or minimized.

3. Assessing service coverage

3.1 Health and environmental services

To obtain an overall assessment of health service coverage for urban communities, examine service provision at the community, primary health unit and hospital levels and investigate service accessibility, affordability and acceptability.

3.1.1 Service provision

There is no direct correlation between physical proximity to health facilities and the delivery of services to or uptake of services by a community. Nevertheless the identification of the various health and environmental services that exist in a community, or are said to be provided for it, is a necessary starting point for assessing service coverage.

Simple enumeration of health facilities, however, is not enough; descriptions of the orientation of service outlets and the service mix are also important. Are services predominantly curative, or primarily promotive and preventive with the necessary curative and rehabilitative provision? Is the orientation and mix of service outlets appropriate to the health needs of the population? Viewed as a comprehensive provision, do all of the health and environmental services available to a community attempt to meet that community's needs for: "the promotion of proper nutrition and an adequate supply of safe water; basic sanitation; maternal and child care, including family planning; immunization against the major infectious diseases; prevention and control of locally endemic diseases; education concerning prevailing health problems and the methods of preventing and controlling them; and appropriate treatment for common diseases and injuries".

It is also important to remember that traditional practitioners are not limited to rural populations. The spectrum of traditional practitioners in an urban community can be considerable, and they may provide the only health services within settlements. Some of these may be "quacks" using conventional medicines in ineffective or harmful ways. By contrast genuine traditional healers, particularly traditional birth attendants, may provide the most available access to health care which many community members have.

3.1.2 Service accessibility

Once identified, services need to be assessed for their accessibility. A variety of factors can limit access by the poor. Financial cost is of increasing importance in many areas. Where cheap and therefore highly utilized services are available, long waiting times may be the problem. Transport costs may limit access to cheap, but distant services. Services that are not responsive to cultural and social sensitivities may render themselves inaccessible.

3.1.3 Service quality

The quality of services which are accessible is an important determinant of service coverage and its effectiveness. In many circumstances, improving the quality of existing services may be the intervention required rather than an attempt to create new services. Some services that are said to exist may be effectively non-existent because of poor quality; in some cases health services may even be detrimental to health!

The availability of staff during working hours, and their attitudes to patients and other clients need to be considered. The adequacy of basic equipment and sundry supplies will influence the quality of many aspects of health care. The supply of drugs, at affordable costs, may determine whether patients attend at all. The quality of the service is closely related to service mix (see section 3.1.1). The knowledge and technical skill of staff are also of vital importance, but are not easily assessed other than by direct methods.

3.1.4 Service organization

The organization of health services is crucially important for promoting equity, and ensuring effectiveness and efficiency in their provision to the community as a whole. Is good use being made of the available resources for the health of the whole community, and not just for privileged groups? Are health and related services planned and provided in a collaborative and coordinated manner? Do mechanisms exist for assuring quality, without unduly limiting opportunities to provide services?

3.2 Social services

Review the other social services available in the community.

Among the urban poor are vulnerable groups for whom a network of educational and social services is necessary, if their lives are to be made more tolerable and so that they can contribute to the community, rather than be a drain on its scarce resources. The range required is much broader than the limited services considered for such groups. The need for educational services for children is usually recognized, even where the current service is non-existent or very restricted. But there is also a need for avenues for informal and functional education, which are at least as important as the availability of primary education.

The only social service provision for many communities consists of community members who have had limited training, for example, as community volunteers. Such volunteers can be of great value, but only if they are consistently supported by professional representatives of the official health, education and other social sectors, including community development.

Other essential social services for urban areas include:

- day-care services for the pre-school children of working mothers;
- rescue and shelter services for abandoned children;
- recreational facilities for children and youths;
- counselling and support services for pregnant girls, and for children and youths involved with drugs, prostitution and other forms of abuse and exploitation;
- rehabilitation services and shelter for elderly people who are no longer self-sufficient.

4. Assessing health policy

Investigate policy and legislation, exploring whether there is the political will to pursue the principles of equity and justice.

The Member States of WHO have endorsed the report of the International Conference on Primary Health Care in Alma-Ata(1), and adopted the Global Strategy for Health for All by the Year 2000. This commitment has not been translated into detailed government policy in all countries, but many have outlined the interest of government with regard to programmes in the health sector. In this context, it is important to realize that the commitment to PHC on the part of governments applies to urban, as well as to rural populations, and that PHC concepts are likewise applicable to urban health systems. Thus a first step in assessing health policy is an investigation of the extent to which the government's endorsement of the PHC strategy has been translated into official policy. The investigation should extend beyond the confines of health policy and enactments alone, to encompass important health-related problems, for example, land rights. It should also include an analysis of budgets, to see whether the promised funds have indeed been allocated to PHC activities.

If a current national health policy document or plan exists it should be examined by those concerned with urban health problems to determine its stance on the urban health system. While it may concentrate on the health of the rural population, it will also have great relevance for urban health planners. There may be a health plan for the municipal authority, or a former plan may contain useful background information on the evolution of local government policy in relation to health.

Many countries have a Public Health Act, often of long standing, and frequently with outdated and unnecessarily restrictive regulations, which may prove a stumbling block for the municipal authority as it attempts to respond to the needs of the rapidly expanding population in the city, and the urban poor in particular. Alternatively there may be clauses which, if implemented, could provide opportunities for new resources to address the most pressing needs. In some countries modern legislation may discriminate in favour of the poor, and make it possible for them to improve their environment.

Reference

1. *Primary health care. Report of the International Conference on Primary Health Care, Alma-Ata, 1978*. Geneva, World Health Organization, 1978 ("Health for All" Series, No. 1).
